Medical Herbalism for Beginners

A Complete Naturopathic Guide to Turning Common Ingredients into Healing Foods and Remedies. There are no Side Effects when Using Natural Antivirals and Antibiotics. How to Make Antibiotic Essential Oils with Herbal Distillation

© Copyright 2022 by **Kevin S. Stevenson**

Medical Herbalism for Beginners

© Copyright 2022 by Kevin S. Stevenson - **All rights reserved**.

This Book is provided with the sole purpose of providing relevant information on a specific topic for which every reasonable effort has been made to ensure that it is both accurate and reasonable. Nevertheless, by purchasing this Book, you consent to the fact that the author, as well as the publisher, are in no way experts on the topics contained herein, regardless of any claims as such that may be made within. It is recommended that you always consult a professional prior to undertaking any of the advice or techniques discussed within.

This is a legally binding declaration that is considered both valid and fair by both the Committee of Publishers Association and the American Bar Association and should be considered as legally binding within the United States.

The reproduction, transmission, and duplication of any of the content found herein, including any specific or extended information, will be done as an illegal act regardless of the end form the information ultimately takes. This includes copied versions of the work, both physical, digital, and audio, unless express consent of the Publisher is provided beforehand. Any additional rights reserved.

Furthermore, the information that can be found within the pages described forthwith shall be considered both accurate and truthful when it comes to the recounting of facts. As such, any use, correct or incorrect, of the provided information will render the Publisher free of responsibility as to the actions taken outside of their direct purview. Regardless, there are zero scenarios where the original author or the Publisher can be deemed liable in any fashion for any damages or hardships that may result from any of the information discussed herein.

Additionally, the information in the following pages is intended only for informational purposes and should thus be thought of as universal. As befitting its nature, it is presented without assurance regarding its prolonged validity or interim quality. Trademarks that are mentioned are done without written consent and can in no way be considered an endorsement from the trademark holder.

Warning

We urge that you visit your doctor or therapist before beginning any treatment.

Kevin S. Stevenson

TABLE OF CONTENTS

INTRODUCTION 5

THE IMMUNE SYSTEM 7

    How does your immune system function? 7
    Elements of the immune system 7
    The Immune System 9
    How to Boost Immune Defences 10
    Natural boosts for the immune system 12
    There are ten things you probably don't know about the immune system. 13

NATURAL ANTIBIOTICS 19

    Natural antibiotics in the kitchen 19
    Other Natural Antibiotics 27

ANTIBIOTIC ESSENTIAL OILS 39

HOW TO MAKE HOMEMADE ESSENTIAL OILS 57

    What you need 57
    Steam Current Distillation 60
    Step-by-step Distillation Process of Essential Oils 63
    Cold Method 68
    How to Prepare an Antibiotic Cream 69

NATURAL ANTIVIRALS 75

    Natural antiviral remedies 75
    Antiviral Essential Oils 87

HOMEMADE ANTIVIRAL PRODUCTS 97

    Antiviral Recipes 98

ANTIVIRAL GASTRONOMY 115

28 Recipes to Fight Flu with Natural Methods 115
CONCLUSION 151

Kevin S. Stevenson

INTRODUCTION

Thank you for purchasing this book and congratulations on doing so. This guidebook is written for anyone who wish to learn how to manufacture natural antibiotic and antiviral essential oils to prevent the spread of bacterial and viral illnesses.

This book provides tried-and-true procedures and tactics for selecting healthy and natural medicines, as well as information on the greatest antibiotics and antivirals that Mother Nature has to offer, as well as the diseases that they combat. Natural treatments are the best example of how nature is the best doctor. Antibiotics were a fantastic discovery, and millions of people have been saved from dreadful diseases since then.

The natural herbs, oils, and foods described in this book have not only shown to be effective antibiotics, but they are also safe, affordable, and do not hurt the body or cause future problems. This book aims to demonstrate, in a straightforward and easy-to-understand manner, which natural antibiotics are the most effective in the treatment of a variety of conditions, ranging from ordinary headaches to viral infections. You'll learn how to strengthen your immune system, as well as how to prevent and treat various forms of viruses, fungus, and bacteria.

Furthermore, you will be shown how to make essential oils using both hot and cold distillation.

The primary goal of this guidebook is to give a useful tool for preparing homemade goods.

When compared to prescription antibiotics, the dangers and side effects of using natural therapies for your health are negligible, if not non-existent. However, we recommend that you visit your doctor before beginning any treatment.

THE IMMUNE SYSTEM

How does your immune system function?

The immune system is made up of a complex network of organs and cells that specialize in protecting the body from illnesses.

Our bodies have a built-in defense mechanism called the immune system, which is essential for protecting us against a variety of foreign chemicals. The majority of these exogenous substances are made up of bacteria, fungus, protozoa, and viruses that are freely circulating in the air. Each of them has chemicals on its surface called antigens, which the immune system recognizes as foreign and attacks.

Elements of the immune system

The immune system consists of a complex "surveillance network" made up of several highly specialized organs and cells, pooled by the lymphatic vessels, and located in various parts of the body that cooperate, each with a specific role, to defend the body and keep it healthy.

Specifically, immune defences are involved:

Lymphatic organs: bone marrow, thymus and lymphatic tissues of the spleen, tonsils, lymph nodes, appendix, Peyer's intestinal plaques.

Cells: white blood cells (leukocytes) circulating in blood and tissue.

Chemical mediators: such as cytokines, proteins that coordinate and perform immune responses, exchanging signals that regulate the level of cellular activity with different organs and tissues.

The lines of defence that activate the immune system against external pathogens can be of three types:

Innate/specific: it acts against any pre-existing external agent in a natural way; immunity therefore does not require previous contact with the pathogen, but its response will be immediate.

Acquired/specific: immunity against the external agent develops slowly and is established following a first contact (both natural and artificial thanks to vaccinations). The resulting antibodies will retain memory for life to act on any further exposure in the future.

Mechanical/chemical: our body activates barriers such as skin, sweat, sebum, acidic pH of the stomach and epithelial membranes covering the respiratory, reproductive and urinary tract, in order to prevent external agents from entering the body.

The Immune System

The various types of cells of the immune system are produced in the bone marrow; this tissue is found inside some bones of the body, particularly large and flat bones such as those that form the pelvis.

The most important cells produced by the immune system are found in the blood and are: phagocytes - i.e. special white blood cells that act "phagocytizing the invaders" for the natural non-specific defence - and lymphocytes - i.e. those white blood cells that modify antibodies against specific pathogens.

There are two classes of lymphocytes:
- **B lymphocytes**: they develop in the bone marrow and are responsible for the production of antibodies, protein molecules capable of recognizing a specific antigen, and bind to them to neutralize them later.
- **T lymphocytes**: they mature in the thymus, an organ located in the chest behind the sternum, and can regulate and coordinate the entire immune system by attacking and destroying altered cells recognized as foreign.

The other components are **white blood cells**, antibodies designed to protect the body from external attacks, but to carry out this task requires the work of the entire immune system, that is:

- **the lymph nodes and lymphatic vessels**: they are part of a circulatory system that carries the lymph, a transparent fluid that contains mainly white blood cells. The lymph is drained into the circulatory stream where it flows into the bloodstream. The lymph nodes are stations within the lymphatic circulation, where the cells of the immune system can reproduce to fight a specific foreign agent. When an infection develops, the lymph nodes will swell;
- **the spleen** is the largest lymphatic organ and is in the upper left abdomen. It is another collection point, where lymphatic cells transport foreign organisms and then fight them.

How to Boost Immune Defences

Our immune defences are naturally vigilant and ready to intervene in case of emergency to defend the body, but it is possible to strengthen it with simple rules.

- Following a balanced diet rich in vitamins and minerals will be of great help to the immune system. Seasonal vegetables and fresh fruit, especially citrus fruits and kiwis, rich in vitamin C, should be consumed.
- moderate sports activity will boost the immune system.
- limiting stress, in fact, is the first cause of the drop in immune defences, as it weakens the white blood cells that react less to external stimuli, leaving our body more exposed to disease.
- a good quality of sleep, with a regular sleep-wake rhythm, will certainly make the immune system more efficient, while lack of sleep can decrease the readiness of the immune defences.
- Avoid smoking. The side effects of smoking are now known to all. It also undermines basic immune defences and increases the risk of bronchitis and pneumonia in all and middle ear infections in children.
- Drink less alcohol. Excessive alcohol consumption compromises the immune system and increases vulnerability to lung infections. Drinking in moderation is a good starting point to increase the body's defences and keep diseases away.
- Consider probiotics. Studies indicate that supplements reduce the incidence of respiratory and gastrointestinal

infections. Fermented milk products have also been shown to reduce respiratory infections in adults and children.

- Sun exposure. Low levels of vitamin D are correlated with an increased risk of respiratory infection. Sunlight triggers vitamin D production by the skin. In summer, exposure of 10-15 minutes is enough to replenish the body with this nutrient. However, above 42 degrees latitude (Boston) from November to February, sunlight is too weak, and few foods contain this vitamin.
- Use lots of garlic. Garlic is a broad-spectrum antimicrobial agent and an immune booster. Since heat deactivates a key active ingredient, add it to foods just before serving.

Natural boosts for the immune system

There are also some aids from nature that are real boosters of the immune system. Foodstuffs include, for example, garlic. The latter, thanks to the presence of allicin, increases the production of cells that fight infection.

Also, worth mentioning are citrus fruits, rich in Vitamin C, a real invigorating factor for the immune system. Not to be forgotten are dried fruit, due to the presence of Vitamin E (known for its antioxidant power, which counteracts the attack of external pathogens), fungi (rich in selenium and beta lucano that stimulate the activation of white blood cells) and salmon (in which Vitamin D is present that counteracts infections of the respiratory tract).

Finally, to strengthen the immune defences, you can use the help offered by natural supplements. These have an invigorating effect on the body's defensive system. Especially when they are composed of the elements that, as seen, act as a real boost for the immune system.

There are ten things you probably don't know about the immune system.

Some scientific curiosities about the invisible and deadly defence apparatus that protects us from external attacks.

1. IS DISTRIBUTED THROUGHOUT THE BODY. The dense surveillance network of the immune system includes a series of organs responsible to produce bi blood cells (spleen, bone marrow, lymph nodes, tonsils, thymus), tissues and circulating cells, connected by lymphatic vessels. The immune cells are also distributed in all the tissues of the body, which they reach thanks to the blood circulation; with such a massive deployment of forces, it is difficult for a pathogen to go unnoticed.
2. ITS FLAGSHIP WEAPONS ARE FOUND IN THE BLOOD. In the arsenal of cells that guard the body, phagocytes and

lymphocytes are the most important ones. The former, which develop in the bone marrow, form a non-specific first line of defence and incorporate foreign molecules into their cytoplasm which, left free to circulate, could create problems. Similar cells with the same functions are also found in very elementary organisms. Pathogens that manage to overcome this first barrier meet a specialized defence: lymphocytes can generate and modify antibodies that recognize specific antigens on the surface of the pathogens, and to neutralize them. Only in vertebrates has this second level of defence developed.

3. WAS FIRST DESCRIBED 2,400 YEARS AGO. The Greek historian Thucydides, describing a plague epidemic in Athens in 430 B.C., noted how people already infected once and surviving did not get sick anymore.

    This principle was exploited in 1796 by the British doctor Edward Jenner to develop the first form of immunization through a vaccine: the smallpox vaccine. Farmers who met forms of bovine or equine smallpox were in fact immune to the human version of the virus.

4. THE SPLEEN IS A NERVE CENTRE. Without the spleen one can live, however, this organ between the stomach and the diaphragm is an important junction for the cells of the immune system. We can imagine it as a sort of giant lymph node where new white blood cells are produced, old ones

are disposed of and those already in circulation are connected.

5. IT ALSO RECRUITS "USELESS" ORGANS. Have you perhaps heard of the appendix as a vestigial organ, so called because for a long time considered a useless remnant of evolution that often becomes inflamed and must be removed. However, it seems that this small structure is important to keep the intestinal bacterial flora balanced and well-matched, especially when the "good bacteria" are in the minority. Some immune cells recently discovered in the appendix, called innate lymphoid cells, help to repopulate the intestine with good bacteria and contain any infection without spreading between tissues.

6. CAN AFFECT SOCIAL INTERACTIONS. The belief that the brain and immune system were isolated and not in communication with each other has been partly disproved by a study published in Nature in 2016. A molecule produced by immune cells in response to infection, gamma interferon, appears to play a major role in the social behaviour of many animals.

In the laboratory, on mice, when this molecule is blocked, animals become less sociable. By restoring it, sociality returns to normal. Social relationships are the main vehicle for the spread of pathogens: the hypothesis is that gamma interferon has encouraged sociality during evolution, helping pathogens to spread but also our immune system to strengthen.

7. SOME OF ITS "KILLER" CELLS BECOME "GOOD" DURING PREGNANCY. The natural killer lymphocytes (the most aggressive cells of the immune system) present in the maternal uterus perform the unsuspected function of nannies in the first weeks of gestation, supporting the foetus with the production of specific growth factors.

8. PAC-MAN CELLS NEUTRALIZE CHILDHOOD TUMORS. Scientists at Stanford University have discovered that a protein expressed on the surface of the cells, called CD47, interacts with macrophages (phagocytes that incorporate, like a Pac-man, pathogens in the first line of defence) sending them a "non-belligerence" signal. Some cancer cells deceive the immune system by producing large amounts of CD47, thus begging the macrophages not to eat them. When this signal is pharmacologically blocked, macrophages can eliminate the cancer cells, reducing the need for therapies with high side effects.

9. CAN BE TRICKED INTO FIGHTING DIABETES. MIT scientists have shown that by encapsulating human pancreatic cells in algae-derived biomaterials and transplanting them to patients with type 1 diabetes, the immune system does not attack them, and their ability to produce insulin remains unchanged.

10. HAS ELEPHANT MEMORY. The immune system can remember an infection even decades later: patients who survived the first Ebola epidemic in the Democratic Republic of Congo are still immune to the infection more than 41 years after infection. This "ability to remember" is due to a small group of lymphocytes that survive even 10 times longer than others, specializing in recognizing the pathogen at the next reappearance.

Medical Herbalism for Beginners

NATURAL ANTIBIOTICS

Antibiotics are substances developed by living organisms or produced in a laboratory that can cause the death of bacteria or prevent their growth.

Like antibiotics, chemotherapy drugs are antibacterial drugs. The difference was originally since chemotherapies are synthetic drugs, whereas antibiotics have a natural origin; the latter come, for example, from the metabolism of fungi (moulds) or certain bacteria (streptomycetes).

Antibiotics represent a constantly evolving pharmaceutical category, so that many natural molecules have been chemically modified to obtain new drugs, called semi-synthetic drugs.

Antibiotics are not effective against viral infections such as colds, flu and certain types of coughs and sore throats.

Natural antibiotics in the kitchen

Our kitchen sometimes offers real natural antibiotics. Let's discover the 5 most common food antibiotics.

When Fleming isolated penicillin in 1928, he paved the way for the world of antibiotics and this allowed the treatment of millions of individuals, thus reducing deaths from infections by an exorbitant percentage.

We certainly owe a great deal to him, but we often ignore the fact that we must be equally grateful to Mother Nature for having given us a plant world so rich in properties; among these is the ability of some plants or foods to be real "natural antibiotics".

Natural antibiotics or simple foods?

When the disease allows it and in order to provide a very valuable aid to the immune system, we can make use of certain types of food that are considered real natural antibiotics!

Plants within them can develop substances as a defence system against microorganisms and bacteria and these substances, when used by humans, consuming those certain plants, have antibiotic action less "aggressive" than drugs, without presenting those side effects so unwelcome to the intestine.

But what are these food antibiotics?
Let's look at the most common natural and food antibiotics in our kitchens.

Garlic

You know the typical "smell" of garlic when the clove is nicked? Well, this unmistakable smell is due to allicin, an active ingredient that makes garlic an excellent natural antibiotic because it can inhibit the action of various bacteria; the same goes for the galicin contained in the bulb.

The garlic plant also contains an essential oil with antibiotic properties composed of allicin, sulphites, diallyl and an enzyme called allinase; known above all for its action of regulating blood pressure, garlic, thanks to its high number of compounds contained within, has the ability to strengthen the immune system in general as well as having a bulb that gives it febrifuge and expectorant properties.

Lemon

The fruit is rich in vitamin C, which is very important in cell defence processes. The ideal would be to take a daily lemon squeeze with a pinch of potassium bicarbonate, which has alkalizing, fungicidal and digestive properties, in hot water (heat kills viruses).

Lemon juice is an antiseptic, bactericide, nervous system tonic and fights bronchitis and arthritis, rheumatism, obesity, hypertension and canker sores. Vitamin C is also present in strawberries, kiwis, potatoes, spinach, broccoli and cherries.

In addition to lemon, citrus fruits are also important.

A valuable source of vitamin C, they help the immune system to protect against disease as well as strengthen the body. They promote the absorption of iron contained in plant foods. They are also perfect for preventing and treating colds and flu, stomatitis, gingivitis and infectious diseases.

Propolis

Did you know that this compound is used by bees to wrap the remains of dead insects so that bacteria do not grow around them?

In propolis are contained various substances such as flavonoids, aldehydes and hydroxy acids; it is precisely the flavonoids that in addition to having anti-inflammatory, antioxidant and haemostatic properties, are very useful to strengthen the immune system. Calcium, nickel, zinc and iron contained in propolis, contribute to the regulation of the immune system and propolis also has an important curative action of respiratory tract diseases.

Onion

Raise your hand if you haven't started to "cry" while cutting an onion to make the fried! The substance attributed to the burning of the eyes is allyl sulphide which, however, has antiseptic properties.

You will be surprised to know that onion, a food rich in vitamins, minerals and other trace elements, as well as helping digestion, is a valuable aid to treat seasonal ailments and has a fluidifying and decongesting effect on the airways, so much so that it might be useful to prepare a syrup based on onion and honey to be taken a couple of times a day.

Oregano

A niche preparation: the essential oil of oregano, which not everyone may know, is an ally of our health.

The undisputed king of our kitchens has active ingredients such as phenols, vitamins and is a good source of mineral salts. Oregano essential oil seems to be one of the most powerful oils with antiseptic properties known to date, and scientific studies have revealed its ability to kill most common bacteria such as staphylococcus. Used in aromatherapy for respiratory problems, this oil is also excellent against cellulite.

Honey

In a scientific study published by researchers at Newport University, it was found that raw honey is one of the best natural antibiotics that can be found in our homes. Scholars have decreed that the property of honey lies in fighting infections on multiple levels while making it more difficult for bacteria to develop resistance.

How does it do this? This is made possible by the combination of polyphenols, hydrogen peroxide and osmotic effect.

In short, in our kitchen are stored foods with beneficial actions on health; we make a fresh, alive and colourful shopping in order to make the most of what nature offers us.

Cinnamon (Cinnamomum zeylanicum)

Cinnamon has antimicrobial and eupeptic properties (facilitates digestion).

It was once used for the treatment of gastrointestinal diseases, bacterial cystitis, vaginitis and oral infections.

Ginger

The scientific community has recognized ginger as a natural antibiotic. Several studies have shown that this root could fight many bacteria.

Cloves

Cloves were generally used to treat teeth. Its extract is effective against many different types of bacteria.

Avocado

The avocado has been considered from a scientific point of view as an important food from which to obtain extracts that can be effective against antibiotic-resistant, such as certain types of staphylococci. The best variety of this fruit from this point of view is the Chilean avocado, one of the characteristic plant species of the South American rainforest, a real treasure trove of biodiversity.

Curcuma

It is an easily available spice with a non-special taste, yet curcuma is a real mine of well-being known since ancient times. Suggestions to make the most of its nutritious principles.

Golden honey: natural remedy for cough and flu

is one of the most widely used traditional remedies to fight viruses, bacteria, strengthen the body's defences when allergy, flu and even cure sore throats. Preparing this remedy is very simple and just have some honey and curcuma.

You simply need them to make it:

- 100 grams of raw honey
- 1 tablespoon of curcuma powder.

Mix the two ingredients well and keep them in a glass jar at room temperature. The expiry date of the product is the same as that of the initial honey.

To have an even more powerful antiviral effect it is recommended to use manuka honey. It has a higher cost, but it is worth it if used in those who tend to take all viruses and colds diseases, who therefore need more support.

How to use Golden Honey

DAY 1: half a teaspoon every hour

DAY 2: half a teaspoon every two hours

DAY 3: half a teaspoon three times a day

Try to keep it in your mouth until completely dissolved. Usually the flu symptoms go away after three days. Many people use this mix as a preventative measure to prevent the onset of the disease.

For respiratory problems such as allergy, cough, sore throat:

FOR ONE WEEK: half a teaspoon 3 times a day. You can also put it in a hot drink.

Contraindications

Curcuma should be avoided by those taking anticoagulant drugs, antacids, chemotherapy. Also, those who have gallbladder problems as curcuma promotes the contraction of the gallbladder muscles. Those with too low a blood pressure should not exaggerate curcuma lowers blood pressure and blood sugar levels.

Green tea

From the leaves of green tea, in addition to the well-known drink, it is possible to obtain a particular polyphenol able to act synergistically with antibiotics in the treatment of bacteria such as Streptococcus and E-coli infections. Green tea is rich in antioxidants believed to be able to perform a preventive action against the appearance of different types of cancer, with reference to the skin.

Neem

From the leaves of the Neem, and from the fruits of this plant, is obtained a powerful curative oil, typically utilized by the traditional Indian medicine, both for alimentary and curative use. To it are attributed antifungal, antibacterial, antiviral and antiparasitic properties. Neem oil for internal use must have been obtained specifically for this purpose and be one hundred percent pure.

Other Natural Antibiotics

Pau d'Arco

Little known in Europe, Pau d'Arco is a plant species of South American origin containing substances considered effective in the treatment of viral, bacterial and fungal infections. It strengthens the immune system and is believed to be able to fight numerous diseases without causing side effects. According to natural medicine experts, it should be used as a replacement for antibiotic drugs for the most common infections.

Olive leaves

The healing properties of olive leaves have been known since the dawn of time to the extent that the Bible speaks of the olive tree as "a tree whose fruits are food and the leaves medicine". The olive leaf is a real chemical laboratory, containing about 250 substances with extraordinary properties including oleanolic acid which is a real natural antibiotic that has shown, in various studies carried out in the laboratory, strong antimicrobial and antiviral activities. Usually taken in the form of an extract, the active ingredients contained in the extract are about 35% more than those contained in extra virgin olive oil. There are also excellent dietary supplements based on olive leaves produced specifically to facilitate their intake.

Aloe Vera

The healing powers of aloe vera have been known for thousands of years: findings dating back 6000 years have been found in Egypt, which demonstrate the use of this plant for both therapeutic and cosmetic purposes.

The plant was commonly used, for example, in folk medicine to treat chronic constipation in a natural way, and there is no traditional medicine, from western to eastern medicine, that does not know its benefits.

Its potency is due to a concentrate of over 160 substances present in it; it also contains 13 different vitamins and minerals, 15 enzymes and many amino acids, as well as many other beneficial properties.

One of the main components that makes aloe so extraordinary is acemannan, which is also found in gingsen and eleuterococcus, which stimulates and balances the immune system, so that it is more reactive against external enemies and falls ill less.

Thyme

As in the case of other aromatic herbs, thyme is also used for phytotherapeutic purposes; it is attributed antiseptic properties at a gastrointestinal level that were known even to the most ancient populations; until the end of the Great War, there were several disinfectants of which it was one of the ingredients.

The antibacterial properties of the plant are attributable to thymol, a simple phenol whose name derives from the fact that it is present in fair quantities in many plants of the genus Thyme.

Modern phytotherapy recommends its use in the treatment of mild urinary and respiratory diseases (in addition to its antiseptic properties, it is also known to have mucolytic and expectorant properties). The forms of use are various: dried drug for herbal tea, dry extract also in association with other plants in capsules or tablets or liquid preparations, fluid extract also in association with other plants for liquid preparations for internal use, essential oil in liquid or semi-solid preparations for skin use and pure oil to be added to bath water.

Nasturtium (Tropaeolum majus)

The leaves and flowers of the nasturtium have antibiotic properties due to their benzyl isocyanate content. Nasturtium has proven effective against several common bacteria. It is used both externally and internally to treat respiratory and urinary tract disorders.

Colloidal silver

Colloidal silver has been known as an effective antibiotic for centuries. In the early 1900s, Alfred Searle, founder of the Searle pharmaceutical company, discovered that it could kill the deadliest pathogens.

Searle claims that applying colloidal silver to his patients was very successful with surprising results. The main advantage is that it is quickly fatal to microbes without having a toxic effect on its host.

Colloidal silver acts as a catalyst and blocks an enzyme that bacteria, fungi and viruses need to live. Infectious agents do not have the ability to develop defence mechanisms against colloidal silver, it kills all pathogenic microorganisms even if resistant to common antibiotics and can no longer use the mechanism of mutation. For more information see All uses of Colloidal Silver.

Burdock (Actium lappa)

This plant has antifungal (antifungal) properties that should be investigated. The preparation of a fresh root extract in alcohol, for example, can be used to treat nail fungi. The plants can be harvested two years after the first seeds have been produced.

Goldenseal

This is one of the most popular herbs sold on the American market and has recently gained a reputation as an immune-boosting herb and as an antibiotic. The American Indians have used goldenseal as a drug for internal inflammatory conditions in the respiratory, digestive, and Genito-urinary tract inflammation induced by allergy or infection.

Pascalitis

This is a type of bentonite clay found only in the mountains of Wyoming. It has remarkable healing powers. When used topically, it is known for its ability to heal wound infections within hours or days, leading to total recovery. The first documented use of Pascalite was in the early 1930s, when a hunter named Emile Pascal set his traps near a mountain lake, where he had noticed a large number of animal tracks; after keeping the clay on his cracked hands, he noticed that it seemed to improve his health after some time. So, he continued to experiment with the substance he discovered in a larger and more extensive number of uses, such as burns, small wounds and infections.

Acacia (Acacia farnesiana, Nilotic)

Some species of this plant have antibacterial properties due to the content of tannins, present in different concentrations. Both leaves and fruits are used.

Ganoderma Lucidum (Reishi)

Ganoderma Lucidum is one of the most tonic and revered herbs in traditional Chinese medicine, Reishi is not only known and consumed to increase longevity and beauty of the body, but also to help find greater concentration, intellectual capacity and spirituality.

For many years, Ganoderma was kept secret from all the people who were not noble and upper class as emperors or kings. When they discovered Ganoderma and its beneficial properties, various people of high society did not allow people of the village or lower class to consume Ganoderma Lucidum, they only had to help cure it and pulverize it to create infusions to serve it to their sovereigns.

Today Ganoderma lucidum is particularly studied because, like other medicinal mushrooms, it can strengthen the body's defences, improving the immune function (in other words, it is an immunostimulant/immunomodulating remedy). Scientific research shows that reishi can even help to prevent and fight certain types of cancer, it also seems for mechanisms of inhibition of angiogenesis and induction of apoptosis (programmed death) of cancer cells.

All degenerative conditions have a chronic inflammatory component, which are caused by alterations and weakness defects of the immune system, Ganoderma works as an adaptogen, an adaptogen is a natural substance found in some rare plants and herbs that protect the body against the effects of stress.

These are nutrients that work at the cellular level to restore, rebalance cells, and re-generate organs.

Adaptogens are not drugs and have no negative side effects, they are not available in the food we eat, they can only be included as supplements, among the natural supplements available adaptogens are considered the most important in their role to improve health and longevity, Ganoderma is considered the most powerful adaptogen ever discovered.

The properties of reishi, however, do not end there, so much so that it is not a bold claim that this oriental fungus is the natural remedy with a thousand virtues, as the mycotherapy experts claim. Its active ingredients, such as first and foremost polysaccharides such as betaglucans and triterpenes such as ganoderic acids, give reishi significant activity in the following areas:

- anti-inflammatory
- adaptogen, against stress, fatigue, weakness and tiredness
- liver protection
- cholesterol regulation
- blood pressure rebalancing
- inhibition of platelet aggregation
- low blood sugar
- decrease in abnormal reactivity of the body in allergies and autoimmune diseases
- antioxidant
- anti-aging
- antibacterial and antifungal (against, among others, Candida albicans and Escherichia coli)
- antiviral (example to influenza and herpes virus).

There seems to be virtually no circumstance in which Ganoderma lucidum cannot help.

Cumin

Cumin (Cuminum cyminum L.) is an herbaceous plant native to Syria. Its seeds are like fennel and aniseed but are smaller and darker. It has digestive properties and is also useful for fighting halitosis.

Cumin has carminative and digestive properties and is a good natural remedy against abdominal swelling and colic.

An excellent herbal tea to drink at the end of a meal to aid digestion can be prepared with the seeds of this precious spice, a pinch of fennel and a little mint, also very useful against coughs.

Chewing cumin seeds would help combat bad breath and stimulate the appetite.

Cumin oil is perfect for massages and wraps, stimulates the circulation and exerts a disinfectant action on the skin.

Cumin is widely used in the cuisine of North Africa, India and the Middle East and is present among the spices of curry and garam masala, a mixture very common in India.

In Morocco it flavours roasted meat, in Mexico it is put in guacamole, in France it flavours certain types of bread while in Spain and Portugal it is found in sausages and vegetable dishes.

Some Dutch and Valle d'Aosta cheeses are also flavoured with cumin.

Eucalyptus (Eucalyptus globulus)

Eucalyptus essence - besides boasting mucolytic and expectorant properties - also has antibacterial properties. Therefore, it can be useful as an antiseptic in case of pharyngitis, bronchitis, otitis and adenitis.

Echinacea (Echinacea)

Echinacea is a plant of the Composite family originating in North America. It is easily found in herbal medicine in the form of mother tincture, dry extracts, infusions and herbal teas.

The leaves are rich in echinacosides and cicoric acid which have antibacterial and antiviral action.

It also contains echinaceine a compound that has anti-inflammatory action. It is rich in flavonoids and caffeic acid that have antioxidant properties.

Echinacea does not produce a real substance with antibacterial action but has adaptogenic and immunostimulant properties that make it useful in the adjuvant treatment of respiratory and low urinary tract infections.

How to use it: infusion and decoction

Pour 1 gram of echinacea roots into a cup of boiling water. Cover the drink and after leaving it to infuse for 10 minutes, strain it with a strainer. This infusion is great for coughs, colds and sore throats," suggests the expert. Alternatively, you can use echinacea to make a decoction. Simply pour into a pot with a lid 750 ml of water, 3 grams of roots and bring to the boil for 5 minutes. After having let the drink rest for 10 minutes, strain it with a strainer and drink it three times a day.

During pregnancy and lactation, echinacea may only be used after consulting your doctor. Echinacea is contraindicated for people with immunodepression and autoimmune diseases.

One of the advantages of echinacea is its versatility. This natural remedy can be used to prevent and treat many small ailments.

Marcela (Achyroclyne saturaoides)

Its flowers in hydroalcoholic extract have a proven antiviral activity. It is a plant little known but widely used in the South Amazon and South America.

Hydraste (Hydrastis canadensis)

Hydraste contains a substance called berberine. This substance has antibacterial properties and can also be useful in the treatment of Candida albicans relapses.

Medical Herbalism for Beginners

ANTIBIOTIC ESSENTIAL OILS

The essential oils consist of a mixture of highly volatile substances and are characterised by an intense odour. For this reason, the components of the essential oils are also called "aromatic".

Essential oils may consist of variable mixtures of substances such as terpenes, alcohols, aldehydes, ketones and esters.

Essential oils extracted from certain types of plants have antibacterial properties. Among these plants, we remember:

- The thyme (Thymus vulgaris).
- The lemon (Citrus lemon).
- Oregano (Origanum vulgare).
- Eucalyptus
- Ginger
- Peppermint (Peppermint x Peppermint).
- Rosemary (Rosmarinus officinalis).
- Curcuma
- Cinnamon

Thyme essential oil

Thyme essential oil is only for external use, never for oral use, because it is so potent that it can damage the mucous membranes. Before applying it to the affected part of the body, it is good to dilute it in a vector or vegetable oil; simple olive oil is also good.

Undiluted thyme essential oil on the skin can cause irritation or inflammation.

It is not recommended if you suffer from high blood pressure or hyperthyroidism.

Lemon essential oil

The properties and uses of lemon essential oil for wellness, beauty and aromatherapy.

Lemon essential oil is obtained from the peels of the lemon and is an essence that boasts many properties: it is antibacterial, improves circulation, stimulates the nervous system. Let's see in detail all the properties and all the uses of lemon essential oil and how to use it for wellness and beauty but also for ecological and kitchen cleaning.

The lemon essential oil is extracted by pressing, distillation or solvent extraction from the lemon peel, the fruit of Citrus lemon. The lemon essence, besides being intensely and pleasantly scented, has numerous properties.

Like most essential oils, lemon essential oil has antibacterial and antiviral properties that make it an excellent ally against coughs, colds and flu states but also to purify domestic environments.

In addition, the essential oil has digestive properties, antioxidant, circulation benefits, strengthens fragile nails and stimulating properties on the nervous system.

Lemon essential oil can be used both internally and externally and can also be spread in environments.

For external use, lemon essential oil should never be used pure but always diluted. It is possible to disperse a drop of essential oil in a teaspoon of aloe vera gel: aloe gel enriched with lemon essential oil is useful to strengthen the capillaries if you suffer from couperose and is an effective natural remedy in case of oily skin with excess sebum and impurities.

Also, externally, lemon essential oil can be used after having diluted a few drops in a vegetable oil, such as sweet almond, sunflower or olive oil: the doses are about 10 drops of lemon essential oil for each tablespoon of vegetable oil. The oil enriched with lemon essential oil can be used to massage legs and buttocks useful to promote circulation, prevent the appearance of capillaries and improve water retention and cellulite.

Internally the lemon essential oil is taken to promote digestion and combat abdominal swelling, adding one or two drops to a teaspoon of honey or a sugar cube: be careful not to exceed the doses.

Lemon essential oil can also be used in cooking to flavour biscuits, cakes and jams.

The external and internal use of lemon essential oil is not recommended during pregnancy, breastfeeding and obviously in case of proven sensitivity to the substances it contains.

Lemon essential oil is also used in aromatherapy: about ten drops in the classic or ultrasound diffuser pleasantly perfume the environment, promote good mood and concentration and improve breathing.

Oregano essential oil

How many times have you used oregano to season a pizza or added to a sauce or plate to flavour it? Maybe you didn't realize it, but at that moment you were taking one of the most powerful antibiotics in the world.

Its essential oil, obtained from the flowering tops, the same ones that in summer are dried after harvesting and then chopped to end up on pizza, contains precious substances useful to treat infections of the respiratory tract and digestive system.

When, at the beginning of the last century, the properties of essential oils began to be studied, oregano was included in the list of 28 major essential oils, those whose antibacterial active ingredients are present in greater quantities than the other essential oils, defined, for this reason, as minor. Oregano is even placed on the podium of the major essential oils, surpassed only by thyme.

Oregano essential oil, with anti-inflammatory, antiviral and antiseptic action, is useful against asthma, dermatitis, cellulite and toothache.

The essential oil of oregano has antiviral and anti-inflammatory properties that make it an effective natural antibiotic. It is mainly recommended:

- In infections: powerful antiseptic, active against all viral forms.
- Asthma, chronic bronchitis: antiseptic and mucus fluidify.
- Difficult digestion: stomachic action, promotes the secretion of gastric juices and digestion. It also has carminative properties, useful in case of meteorism and flatulence.
- Dermatosis, mycosis and psoriasis: healing and germicidal properties.
- The essential oil of oregano is extracted by the method of steam distillation of the flowering tops harvested in summer. The essential oil of oregano is amber-coloured and has a liquid consistency.

- It is used in various ways, within suffumigias to treat colds, bronchitis and coughs.
- For local use it can be used in the treatment of skin blemishes such as acne and blackheads.
- Massaged into the skin after an insect bite it relieves itching and possible redness.
- Oregano essential oil has a relaxing effect on the muscles if added in the water of a warm bath.
- For external use it can be massaged onto the muscles to relieve pain and decontract tired muscles. In this case, it should be diluted in a carrier oil such as sweet almond oil.
- Friction on the scalp eliminates lice and helps slow down hair loss by stimulating regrowth.
- It is an excellent anti-cellulite if massaged on the affected parts of the skin.
- It is an excellent room deodorant and helps keep ants and other insects away thanks to its repellent effect.

Contraindications

Oregano essential oil is contraindicated in children, during pregnancy and breastfeeding. In high doses it is irritating and toxic to the skin. It must always be used diluted.

Eucalyptus essential oil

Eucalyptus essential oil is a truly precious natural remedy. There are different types of eucalyptus essential oil.

The most widely used is eucalyptus essential oil obtained from the leaves of Eucalyptus globolus, which is considered particularly effective for colds and respiratory disorders affecting the bronchi. Eucalyptus essential oil has analgesic and antibacterial properties. In case of colds and respiratory problems it contributes to the expulsion of catarrh. It is considered beneficial both for skin care and the respiratory system. In general, its perfume gives well-being and recalls positive sensations. A characteristic that makes its use in aromatherapy popular. The diffusion of eucalyptus essential oil in the air makes it possible to combat the germs present in the home during periods of illness (e.g. flu and colds).

It helps to decongest the respiratory tract. It has a refreshing power that makes it useful in case of fatigue and exposure to high temperatures, for example during the summer season. It can help the body to regulate the temperature in case of fever. Used for massages, it can help improve blood circulation and promote vasodilation.

It can also help fight infections affecting the gastrointestinal tract, for example by massaging the abdomen in case of dysentery. It is considered useful for fighting lice. Massages with eucalyptus essential oil can be beneficial for those suffering from neuralgia.

It has antiviral, pain-relieving and anti-inflammatory properties. Those who know plantar reflexology can find benefit in massaging the essential oil of eucalyptus on the points of the sole of the foot corresponding to the area to be treated. Eucalyptus essential oil can also be indicated in cases of acne and labial herpes. It is used for the preparation of mouthwashes suitable for disinfecting the oral cavity. Finally, it's refreshing, and antibacterial properties make it suitable during sauna and Turkish bath.

Eucalyptus essential oil contains active ingredients that make it a powerful antibacterial agent. It is commonly used to treat skin infections and to inhibit inflammation. Its use can also be useful in home care.

In case of colds and to clear the stuffy nose, you can use eucalyptus essential oil. Two or three drops are enough in the preparation of suffumigias with a litre of boiling water and a teaspoon of baking soda. Or you can pour a drop on a handkerchief and breathe to obtain a refreshing effect. It is considered an essential oil with a powerful balsamic and decongestant power, to be applied by friction on the chest.

The use of eucalyptus essential oil is recommended for massages in case of muscle pain, fatigue and accumulation of lactic acid. You can apply a few drops of eucalyptus essential oil - better if diluted in vegetable oil, for example coconut or almond oil - to the areas affected by muscle pain by practicing a gentle massage, always heading towards the heart. So, in the case of the legs, from the bottom upwards, from the feet towards the pelvis.

WARNINGS

Eucalyptus essential oil is considered unsuitable for children. Always keep it out of their reach. Never use any essential oil in children under 3 years of age, unless instructed to do so by an expert, because although essential oils are natural substances, they are very potent and can cause unwanted reactions. Always buy pure essential oils - in an herbalist's shop, in a pharmacy or on the internet from trusted websites - and that are suitable for aromatherapy and skin application.

Ginger essential oil

Among the essential oils, ginger is certainly in a less prominent position than, for example, tea tree oil, essential oil of lavender, mint, lemon, eucalyptus or thyme, which are much better known and used.

In fact, like its "companions", ginger essential oil is also a natural remedy with excellent properties and useful in various circumstances.

Ginger essential oil as well as fresh rhizome is an excellent anti-nausea remedy. The active ingredients contained in it make it possible to limit the discomfort caused by different types of nausea: those caused by travelling by car, train, ship, plane, etc., but also post-operative nausea, due to the taking of medicines as well as pregnant ones.

This essential oil has pain-relieving and anti-inflammatory as well as antiseptic properties and is therefore one of the natural remedies useful to keep germs and bacteria away, preventing certain diseases thanks to the disinfection of the air or the environment. Much appreciated also because it counteracts stagnant liquids in the body and reactivates the circulation as well as a stimulating remedy for the immune system.

Another interesting property of ginger essential oil is that it includes the psychological and emotional sphere. Its aroma is in fact a mood tonic and therefore predisposes to optimism and mental clarity.

Some benefits of this essential oil can finally be used for the care and well-being of body and hair. For example, ginger essential oil can help to improve hair regrowth and is a natural anti-dandruff agent.

Peppermint essential oil

The essential oil of peppermint is very appreciated for its ability to free the respiratory tract but is also very useful for those who study or work as it promotes concentration and relieves stress.

Peppermint essential oil is effective against bacteria but also against fungi and dust mites. Diffused in environments purifies the air, while a few drops between the sheets or on cushions and sofas prevent the proliferation of mites.

To free the respiratory tract spread the essence of mint is useful when you have difficulty breathing. If you are away from home, you can put two drops on a handkerchief and breathe whenever you want to clear your nose. Alternatively, you can make suffumigias by pouring 4/5 drops of essential oil into boiling water and then breathe by covering your head with a towel and closing your eyes.

The strong smell of mint helps concentration, tones body and mind and helps to keep fatigue, stress and nervousness away. The best way to enjoy these properties of mint essence is to spread it in rooms when needed but you can also use it diluted in a vegetable oil for a relaxing massage.

Many people successfully use mint essential oil in case of headaches. To take advantage of its pain-relieving power, just a few diluted drops are enough to massage gently on the temples, spread the essence in the rooms or smell it directly from the bottle. Mint is also excellent for fighting rheumatic or muscular pains, in this case it is better to choose massages.

Mint oil is one of the most suitable to free the respiratory tract in case of cold or sinusitis. It can be spread in the environment, inhale directly from a handkerchief, use it to take a relaxing hot bath or even to make suffumigies.

Few essential oils give a great feeling of freshness like peppermint oil. This essence is particularly suitable for refreshing and disinfecting the oral cavity as well as fighting halitosis, not surprisingly it is very often found as an ingredient in toothpastes and mouthwashes.

Mint oil is a strong digestive stimulant, that's why in aromatherapy it is often recommended to solve gastrointestinal problems and fight the feeling of nausea, even the one due to car sickness. However, nausea cannot be used during pregnancy.

The smell of peppermint essential oil does not like insects, so it can be useful to spread it during the period when there are many mosquitoes to keep them away from the places where you stay.

Rosemary essential oil

The essential oil of rosemary is obtained from Rosmarinus Officinalis, a plant of the Labiatae family. Known for its stimulating and purifying properties, it is useful as a cardiotonic and anti-cellulite.

Properties and benefits of rosemary essential oil

Stimulant, on the nervous system if inhaled, gives energy, promotes concentration and improves memory, especially during periods of strong pressure for intellectual activities. If used in the morning it performs a general toning action; it dissolves and stimulates our emotional components, gives courage and strengthens the will. A true enemy of illusions, it teaches us to look away and clearly perceive the nuances of life.

Cardiotonic, this essence has a marked effect on the heart, for this reason it is indicated in cases of asthenia, low blood pressure, weakness and tiredness, even mental.

Purifying, 2-3 drops in half a teaspoon of honey, it stimulates biliary drainage and digestion, removes waste and dissolves stagnation from the body supporting the detoxifying activity of the liver.

Anticellulite, it is used as an ingredient in cosmetic products and mud against cellulite or localized adiposity, by virtue of its lipolytic action (dissolves fats), stimulates peripheral circulation and drains the lymphatic system.

Anti-inflammatory, if massaged locally diluted in sweet almond oil, it relieves joint and muscle pain, dissolves uric acid and crystals that harden the epidermal tissues forming oedemas, swelling and water retention.

Astringent, it has a tonic, antiseptic and purifying effect on the skin. It is useful in the treatment of acne and dark skin spots. For these properties it is also used as an ingredient in lotions and shampoos for oily hair, with dandruff and to combat hair loss, as it stimulates circulation, promotes tissue oxygenation and hair regrowth.

Use and practical advice on rosemary essential oil

Environmental diffusion: 1 cc of rosemary essential oil, for each square meter of the environment in which it spreads, by means of an essential oil burner or in the water of the humidifiers of the radiators to refresh and deodorize the air and promote concentration.

Anti-cellulite oil: Dilute 5 - 10 drops in oil 100 ml of sweet almond oil and friction, cellulite water retention, bad fat circulation localized on thighs and buttocks. **Toning bath**: Dilute 10-15 drops of essence in a tub of water to restore calm and neutralize tension, fight stress and in the presence of rheumatism, muscle pain, arthritis, contusions and sciatica.

Anti-fall shampoo: pour a few drops in a neutral shampoo and proceed with washing in case of weak, fragile, greasy hair and with dandruff, alopecia. At the end, on damp hair, a few drops rubbed on the scalp will prove to be a panacea.

Contraindications.

Rosemary essential oil is not irritating, but should always be used diluted, and not for long periods. Pay attention to the quantities because in high doses it can be toxic when used internally. Contraindicated in pregnancy, in epileptics and for children.

Curcuma essential oil

You can prepare curcuma oil for both cosmetic and food use. It is prepared by mixing 3 tablespoons of curcuma to 500 ml of extra virgin olive oil in a hermetically sealed jar. Close and let it macerate for a week. Shake the jar once a day and on the eighth day pour it all into a bottle without moving the curcuma left on the bottom. Curcuma oil is more powerful than curcuma alone because it makes the active ingredients more bioavailable.

Cinnamon essential oil

Cinnamon essential oil is obtained from Cinnamomum zeylanicum, a plant of the Lauraceae family. Known for its antiseptic and invigorating properties, it is useful against diarrhea, coughs and colds.

<u>Properties and benefits of cinnamon essential oil</u>

Invigorating, if inhaled, promotes creativity and inspiration. It warms the heart and gives an enveloping feeling of "home", helps in cases of inner coldness, depression, loneliness and fear.

Antiseptic, like all essential oils, it exerts a powerful broad-spectrum antibacterial action. In internal use, 2 drops diluted in a little honey, is useful in case of diarrhea caused by intestinal infections and parasites. For this property is also an effective remedy against flu, in the presence of coughs and colds.

Carminative a few drops in almond oil, massaged on the abdomen promotes the elimination and absorption of intestinal gas and helps the digestive process.

Stimulates the nervous system, with mild aphrodisiac effect, accelerates the exhalation and heartbeat.

Practical uses and advice on cinnamon essential oil

Environmental diffusion: 1 cc for every square metre of the environment in which it spreads, by means of an essence's burner, or in the humidifiers of the radiators.

Suffumigi in a bowl of boiling water put 8-10 drops of cinnamon essential oil, cover the head with a towel and inhale deeply with the nose for 3 minutes, interrupt briefly and resume inhaling. Continue in this way until the water releases steam.

Massage oil: in 200 ml of sweet almond oil put 20 drops, massage, 2-3 times a day, the belly in case of slow digestion, in the presence of intestinal gas and diarrhea.

Contraindications

At high doses inhalation can lead to a convulsive state. On the skin it is a rubefactor, it causes a strong heating of the area, so its use requires caution. The internal use should be done for a short time, to avoid sensitization of the mucous membranes. It is contraindicated in pregnancy, breastfeeding and in children. Before any type of intake, consult your herbalist.

Medical Herbalism for Beginners

Kevin S. Stevenson

HOW TO MAKE HOMEMADE ESSENTIAL OILS

Essential oils, i.e. all the aromatic substances responsible for the scent of plants, have been known and used since ancient times.

Over the centuries, there has been an alternation of glory and oblivion, the latter essentially as a result of the progress of chemistry and synthetic molecules. But as early as the 1990s, essential oils have once again become the object of investigation and there has been an increasing use of what is known as Aromatherapy.

This term refers to the use of essential oils in order to improve the quality and sensation of health and well-being on a physical, emotional and mental level.

The extraction of essential oils from aromatic plants is certainly a fascinating process, which requires an in-depth study of the plants, but can also be carried out within the home in extreme simplicity.

What you need

- A distiller
- gas or electric cooker

- water
- aromatic plants with a high content of essential oils (Mint, Lavender, Thyme, Rosemary, Savory, Sage, etc.).

It is not necessary to have a chemical laboratory, as this can work on your kitchen stove.

Of course, you need to have the raw material available, i.e. the plants to be distilled: about 2 kg of fresh plant, harvested in the so-called balsamic time, the period in which the plant reaches the maximum concentration of active principles.

In small distillers, even a small quantity of aromatic plants is enough, and it is therefore essential that they have a high concentration of essence in their plant cells, otherwise not even a drop would be extracted. For example, by distilling Lavender, Rosemary, Thyme, Sage, Mint, Savory, Lippia and Eucalyptus, it will be possible to obtain up to 10 ml of essential oil, completely produced by you.

The essential oils are extracted by **steam distillation**, a technique that exploits the steam produced by boiling water that, passing through the plant placed in the distiller, drags with it the aromatic molecules contained in the plant cells. These molecules are very light, small and therefore easily vaporized. The water vapour and the volatile molecules continue their path passing inside a condenser and both return to the liquid state.

By their nature, essential oils are lighter than water and will therefore float on top of the so-called aromatic water (the vapour returned liquid in which micro-drops of essential oil are dispersed, giving it the typical fragrance of the distilled plant). The two liquids being immiscible from each other are easily separable using a simple separating funnel.

The products obtained are:
- Pure essential oil
- Aromatic water also called hydrolate.

Aromatic water is not a "waste" product but it is the second product of the distillation of which it can be widely used, from water for ironing to tonic to cleanse the face but also to water our plants with water enhanced with an important antiseptic power. Remember that the freshly distilled essential oil does not always have a pleasant scent, because it needs a period of maturation (a few weeks), in which it must be left to rest.

Storage

The essential oil produced is a very delicate substance that can easily alter and become rancid, thus losing its natural scent and developing substances that can also be harmful; therefore it is important to store them in dark glass bottles away from direct light and heat sources.

As we well know, the use of essential oils takes place by drops; their use, in fact, must be limited to small quantities since these substances are highly concentrated and rich in active molecules, many of which can also have toxic effects. Therefore, when using them, it is always necessary to go carefully and seek advice from experts.

Steam Current Distillation

Steam distillation is a technique that allows essential oils to be extracted from the fabric of the plant by transporting them by water vapour.

This extraction technique is based on the physical property of the essential oils to be volatile, i.e. easily vaporized and dragged by water vapour.

The aromatic plant to be distilled can be used both in the fresh state and in the dry state.

Preference is given to the fresh plant, harvested at the right time of day and in its balsamic time, i.e. when the concentration of active principles inside the plant is maximum.

The time elapsing between the harvesting of the plant and its distillation must be as short as possible, in order to avoid the alteration and dispersion of the essential oil during storage.

The plant, before being placed inside the distiller, must be previously cleaned from insects, material not suitable for distillation and weeds.

The passage of steam, generated by the boiling of water, through the plant material, makes the cell walls more permeable, up to the point of breaking and releasing the essence, which, being volatile, is vaporized.

The mixture of water vapour/essence is condensed in a coil cooled by a water recirculation and returned to the liquid state, separating into essential oil and distilled water.
The essential oil is deposited on the surface because it has a lower density than water.

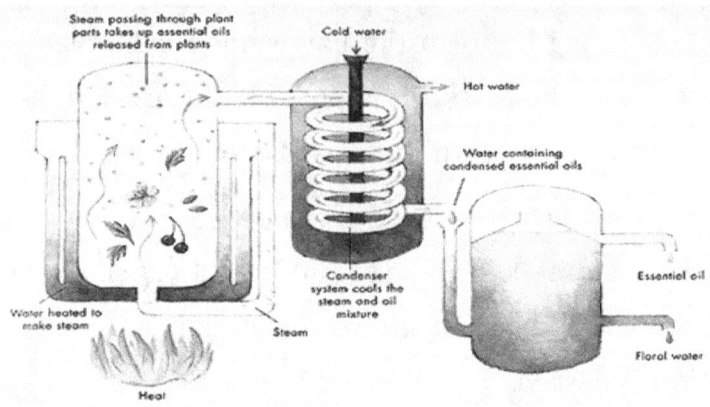

The essence obtained, before being used, must undergo a purification process that consists of eliminating unnecessary, irritating and organoleptically unpleasant components.

The water collected is an aromatic water because it contains a small percentage of essential oil dissolved in it and which gives it the scent of the plant placed to distil.

It can be used in cosmetics, in the kitchen, as water for ironing to perfume laundry.

The essential oils obtained by distillation are widely used in perfumery, in the preparation of phyto-cosmetics, in the food industry as aromatizes and for their therapeutic action in Aromatherapy.

Step-by-step Distillation Process of Essential Oils

As mentioned earlier, essential oils are highly concentrated oils that are extracted from aromatic plants, such as oregano and rosemary. There are about 700 different types of plants that contain useful essential oils and numerous extraction methods - the most common is distillation. Although they are expensive products to buy, their home distillation is quite cheap.

Choose when to collect the material. The amount of oil in a plant depends on the stage of the plant's life cycle, so it is essential to harvest each plant species at the right time. You need to do some research to figure out when to collect the plants you want to distil. For example, lavender should be taken when about half of the flowers have withered. Rosemary, on the other hand, should be picked when it is in full bloom.

Harvest the plants correctly. You need to find out about harvesting techniques, just like you did to know the right timing. By handling the material carelessly, harvesting the wrong parts of it or even just at the least indicated time of day, you can reduce the quantity and quality of the essential oils. For example, you only need to use the apical flowering of rosemary to extract the oil. Throw the rest of the plant away or use it in another way.

Most essential oils are contained in the plant's oil glands, veins and trichomes - all very fragile structures. If you disturb or break them during harvesting, you will get less oil. Handle the plant material with great care and as little as possible.

Dry the plant material. This reduces the amount of oil in each plant, but it greatly increases the amount you can extract from each batch because it allows you to process more material at a time. Drying should be done slowly and away from direct sunlight. Plants you can buy, such as lavender and mint, are sometimes left to dry in the field for about a day after harvest.

The ideal drying method varies depending on the plant, but in general you should avoid exposing the plant material to excessive heat. The process carried out in the shade or even in a dark room minimizes oil loss.

Make sure that the plants do not get wet before distillation, processing them as soon as possible after drying them.

You can also decide not to dry them if you prefer to skip this step.

Distillation

Pour the water into the tank or the alembic still. If you are using handcrafted equipment, the tank is the pressure cooker. Use clean water; in theory, it should be filtered or distilled and with as little limescale as possible. If you bought a distiller, follow the manufacturer's instructions. In any case, make sure you use enough water to complete the process. Depending on the type and amount of plant material, distillation could last from thirty minutes to six hours or more, depending on the boiling water.

Add the plant material to the water. Try to fill the tank completely. If you have enough water that does not overflow during boiling, you can also compact the plants. Make sure, however, that they do not obstruct the passage of steam through the valve on the lid of the pressure cooker.[7] Leave about 5 cm of margin.

You must not break or prepare the plants in any other way, otherwise you will lose some of the oil contained.

Bring the contents of the pressure cooker to the boil. Seal the lid so that steam can only escape through the hose that you have connected to the valve. Most plants release the oil when it reaches 100 °C - the normal boiling point of water.

Check the still. After some time, the distillate should start to flow through the condenser and separator. The process should not require any intervention on your part, but you should make sure that the water in the pressure cooker does not run out. Depending on the duration of the distillation, it may be necessary to change the water in the cooling system. When the glass tube heats it, you must replace it with cold water or add ice to allow the condensation process to continue.

Filter the oil you have collected (optional). Once the distillation is finished, you can decide to filter the product through a cheesecloth or similar fabric, cotton and dry. Make sure the cloth is dry and clean, as residues of detergent and dirt can contaminate the oil.

Don't feel disappointed if you only get a very small amount of essential oil from a lot of plant material. The percentage yield varies depending on the species of plant.

Pour the oil quickly into a container for storage. Most essential oils last at least one or two years, but others only last for a very short time. To be able to use the oil for as long as possible, keep it in a dark glass bottle or stainless-steel container. Use a clean funnel to decant the oil and make sure the container is intact before proceeding. Finally, place the oil in a cool, dark place.

Decide what to do with the hydrosol. The material left in the separator is called hydrosol and is the distilled water into which the scent of the plant has been infused.

Some of these hydrosols, such as rose or lavender, can also be used on their own.

If you don't want to keep it, you can pour it back into the still for immediate distillation of the next batch of plant material or you can throw it away.

Tips

Essential oils are extremely concentrated, and it is generally recommended to dilute them in a carrier oil before applying them to the skin. The most widely used is almond oil, but others can also be used. Vector oils should be added during the bottling phase or mixed with pure essential oils just before application. Usually, the second method is preferred, because in some cases it is useful to have the pure oil; in addition, the vector oil is preserved for less time.

Warning

- ✓ Most essential oils should not be ingested, especially in pure form. Many should also be diluted for topical application. In addition, some of these extracts are toxic.
- ✓ Most flowers should be distilled immediately after harvesting, skipping the drying stage.
- ✓ Do not distil a batch of plant material for too long (check the advice for the specific plant); even if this way you can obtain larger quantities of oil, there is a risk of contaminating it with unwanted chemical compounds.
- ✓ If the plant is of organic origin, this does not mean that it has not been treated with pesticides or fertilisers, but that the products used are not of synthetic origin. However, some organic fertilisers and pesticides are more toxic than synthetic ones. Try to get the material from a farmer in the area who can give you all the information about his cultivation techniques.

- ✓ When drying the plant, you should take care that the material does not become contaminated with soil, dust or other substances, because the quality of the oil would be affected and the oil itself could become unusable.

Cold Method

To prepare the essential oil at home, first choose a vegetable oil as a base, such as olive oil, almond oil (more suitable to be applied on the skin) or wheat germ oil. It is also important to use only organic herbs or flowers without pesticides. Collect, preferably early in the morning, a 250 ml cup of fresh herbs and flowers. Put the leaves and flowers collected, washed and well dried with absorbent paper in a plastic bag; close it and lightly crush it with a wooden pestle or rolling pin. This operation serves to release the oil from the aerial parts of the plant. Immediately afterwards put them in a large glass jar, with a large mouth and cork, together with 250 ml of the vegetable oil of your choice. Place the jar in a warm place not in direct contact with the sun for 24-48 hours, during which time the plants will give off their aroma. Then filter with the help of cotton gauze. To strengthen the fragrance and the concentration of the oil you can add other herbs and flowers treated in the same way as described above, leave to rest for another 24-48 hours and filter again.

How to Prepare an Antibiotic Cream

Garlic Cream

To get all the benefits of garlic, you must eat it raw, as it loses 90% of its properties when cooked. Allicin, the active ingredient responsible for the medicinal effects of garlic, is released when it is chopped or crushed.

Garlic is widely used throughout the world, but not everyone is aware of its medicinal properties. In this article we would like to show you how to prepare a garlic antibiotic cream.

For many centuries natural medicine has used garlic in the treatment of various ailments because this bulb has properties that can fight infections, fungi, bacteria and help to cleanse and purify the blood.

The magnificent properties of garlic are obtained once the bulb is crushed, as this procedure releases a substance called allicin which is the basis of many drugs produced by pharmaceutical companies.

Uses that can be made of garlic

- For almost all injuries, you can crush the garlic directly on the wound. This procedure will relieve the pain and prevent the formation of an infection as allicin enters the bloodstream.

- If ingested, garlic also helps to generate beneficial bacterial flora and counteracts the negative effect of pills and tablets in the stomach.
- In the case of infections caused by fungus, such as athlete's foot for example, it is useful to apply garlic paste to the feet, like a cream, and then cover them with a pair of socks. It is advisable to use these clothes exclusively for the treatment of the ailment in question and to throw them away once the treatment is finished.
- Likewise, garlic paste is useful against rashes, for example in the case of acne or herpes, both oral and genital.
- You can experience another of the benefits of garlic by simply rubbing it on your chest to relieve colds or pneumonia. If, on the other hand, you rub it on the nasal cavities you can relieve sinusitis and rhinitis.
- Finally, garlic is a powerful analgesic and antibiotic when used for ears, once rubbed on a swab.

To make this wonderful antibiotic cream with multi-purpose garlic you just must remember the "three x three" rule.

You need three ingredients, namely virgin coconut oil, extra virgin olive oil and fresh garlic. To prepare the ointment you will need three tablespoons full of each of these ingredients.

Procedure to follow

Heat the coconut oil over low heat, add the olive oil and stir evenly.

When the mixture is hot and homogeneous, add the chopped garlic, fry it and then remove the pot from the heat.

Put the mixture in a blender, or pound it in a mortar or coffee grinder.

Filter it all and pour it into a jar.

You might also be interested: Calm the pain with ginger and olive oil...

That's it! Now you have your own personal antibiotic ointment and analgesic.

Keep it in the fridge and don't forget that the ointment only keeps its properties intact for two weeks.

Once prepared, the ointment will have a white colour and consistency like milk. However, it will gradually become softer and thicker.

After a few hours in the refrigerator, you will discover that it will have increased its consistency and become a kind of cream and in this way, it will be easy to spread.

As soon as it is prepared, the ointment will have a white colour and a consistency like that of milk. However, little by little it will become softer and thicker.

After a few hours in the refrigerator, you will find that it will have increased its consistency and become a kind of cream and in this way, it will be easy to spread.

Thyme Cream

The thyme cream is prepared with balsamic essential oils that make it a useful remedy in case of cold, cough, fever, muscle aches and skin problems.

Thyme cream is a cosmetic or medicinal product that contains balsamic essential oils useful in case of cold, fever, muscle fatigue and skin problems.

Generally, the type cream is prepared using essential oils of thyme, eucalyptus and mint, to which essences of lavender, orange, camphor, tea tree and others can also be added.

The use of thyme cream for colds, coughs or fevers is very simple, as it is enough to massage the cream onto the chest and back once or twice a day, preferably before going to sleep.

Likewise, in case of pain, tears or muscle fatigue, you can get relief from thyme cream massages on the affected area.

In case of acne, thyme cream can be used for pimples, especially if they are spread on the back or body, spreading a thin film of product over the areas to be treated.

Although thyme cream contains antibacterial essential oils, it is not recommended for vaginal candida, unless it is specifically formulated for intimate areas.

Given the content of essential oils, it is preferable to consult your doctor before using thyme cream during pregnancy, while breastfeeding or on children.

Thyme cream is easily available on the market, in herbal shops and natural cosmetics stores, but it is also possible to prepare an equally effective thyme ointment at home.

Preparing thyme cream at home is really very simple because it has few ingredients and takes just a few minutes.

Ingredients

- 50 drops of sunflower oil
- 6 drops of beeswax
- 20 drops of thyme essential oil
- 10 drops of eucalyptus essential oil
- 5 drops of mint essential oil

Preparation

Melt the beeswax in a bain-marie in sunflower oil, stirring occasionally.

When the mixture appears liquid and homogeneous, pour it into a clean, dry, lidded glass jar. Allow to cool, add the essential oils and stir slightly, before closing the container.

Allow to cool for at least 24 hours before using thyme ointment,

The product can be kept from one to three months away from direct sources of light and heat: it is advisable to indicate on the packaging the date of preparation and the list of ingredients.

NATURAL ANTIVIRALS

Antivirals are drugs whose use is intended to fight numerous viral infections or to provide protection, usually for a short period, against the infection itself. They act by inhibiting one of the various phases of the virus replication cycle (absorption and penetration of the virus into the host cell; transcription and translation of the viral genome; assembly and maturation of virions, i.e. complete viral particles). They can have therapeutic and preventive action.

There are different types of antiviral drugs, each one specific to combat a particular type of virus.

Natural antiviral remedies

There are some herbs and natural products that can increase the release of interferon. This means improving the immune response against viruses.

Let's start with the most powerful and most studied class of natural remedies: medicinal mushrooms

Medicinal Mushrooms

Medicinal mushrooms are among the most powerful weapons that nature has put at our disposal against the Virus threat!

They act precisely as interferon activators, especially for the IFN-γ category. The action is carried out by the polysaccharide component that some of them contain (β-glucans).

The polysaccharides of fungi enhance the immune response, which becomes faster and more effective in responding to the aggression of the virus.

These substances bind to specific membrane receptors located on the surface of phagocytic cells and NK (Natural Killer) cells, stimulating their immune response to a viral infection.

The fungi that possess this peculiar function are:

Cordyceps synesis

Cordyceps synesis is a fungus of the millenary Chinese tradition, used for centuries as an adaptogenic fungus, to strengthen the immune system and for its ability to improve mental, physical and sexual performance.

It also has strong antiviral properties.

As evidenced by several studies thanks to the action of cordycepin, Cordyceps can inhibit viral replication through the inhibition of reverse transcriptase. In addition, it is ideal for the regulation of interferon production (IFN-γ).

The Ganoderma Lucidum

Ganoderma Lucidum, also known as Reishi, is probably the most famous fungus of Traditional Chinese Medicine.

It is also considered a powerful adaptogen, able to reduce inflammatory states and improve the immune response to viruses, bacteria and parasites.

As the studies show, Ganoderma stimulates the lymphocytic subpopulations responsible to produce IL-2, increasing the activity of cytotoxic T lymphocytes and stimulating the production of IL-1. In general, the polysaccharide fraction exerts a stimulation effect on leukocytes, monocytes, macrophages, Natural Killer cells and LAK cells. All these actions are responsible for the antiviral and bactericidal activity. In addition, it is an excellent regulator of interferon production (IFN-γ).

Other fungi with similar actions are Agaricus, Shiitake and Maitake.

How to take the medicinal mushrooms

As experts advise, it is good to associate the intake of medicinal mushrooms with the consumption of vitamin C, better if it comes from natural sources, such as lemon juice, or rose hip tea.

Vitamin C promotes better absorption of beta-glucans, active ingredients with antiviral action.

A preventive consumption of 2 g per day is recommended. From 4g to 8g per day in case the infection is already present.

Contraindications

Both Reishi and Cordyceps synesis are safe products, catalogued by Traditional Chinese Medicine as "superior herbs", a category of herbs that can be taken daily for a lifetime without side effects.

However, since they are mushrooms, it is best to avoid them if you are allergic to mushrooms or yeasts. Furthermore, they are not recommended for people who have undergone an organ transplant.

Licorice

Licorice is an unusual medicine. It is powerful antiviral, moderately antibacterial, moderately immunostimulant, and vigorously synergistic.

Preparation and dosage

One of the fundamental things to remember when using licorice is that the higher the glycyrrhizin content, the greater its antiviral activity. If you use it as an antiviral, therefore, it should not be licorice deglycyrrhizinase (DGL).

Choose roots at least three years old (four if you use G. uralensis). The glycyrrhizin content of younger roots is much lower than that of older roots.

Licorice infusion

Dissolve 1 or 2 teaspoons of root powder in 250 ml of water, let the mixture simmer for 15 minutes without lid, then strain it. Drink up to 3 cups per day. One cup every two hours for acute phase treatment.

Licorice decoction

In Japan, the traditional preparation is as follows: 6 g of root powder diluted in 500 ml of water. Bring the mixture to a boil and continue cooking over moderate heat, without lid, until the liquid has reduced to half. At this point the liquid will be rather mucilaginous; then add enough water to bring the volume to one litre. Drink the decoction throughout the day.

Side effects and contraindications

Liquorice is generally safe; it is not toxic even in high doses. However, using it for a prolonged period can give rise to a number of side effects. This can also happen simply by drinking licorice infusion regularly for several years. Side effects can be important, especially in the elderly and pregnant women.

Properties of licorice

Licorice is a powerful virus-static remedy, even vaguely virucide.

Also, licorice is:

- Analgesic
- Antibacterial
- Antihemolytics
- Anti-inflammatory
- Antioxidant
- Antispasmodic
- Anti-stress
- Anti-cough
- Antitumoral
- Antiulcer
- Cardioprotective
- Cytoprotective
- Contrasts hyperglycemia

- Emollient
- Hepatoprotective
- Expectorant
- Estrogenic
- Immunomodulant
- Immunostimulant

Antiviral effectiveness

Licorice is a broad-spectrum antiviral, active against a wide range of viruses due to its multiple mechanisms of action. It strongly impedes the formation of pores in cell membranes, which is one of the strategies implemented by certain viruses to penetrate cells. This inhibition slows down viral infection and, in some cases, prevents it altogether. With other viruses, it has a directly virucide action and with others it stimulates the immune system of the host to attack the invading agent in a highly specific way.

Ginger

Ginger is a respectable antiviral only if its fresh rhizome is used. It is not when using dried root. More specifically, the juice of the fresh rhizome.

Preparation and dosage

If you use ginger as an antiviral, the fresh juice is unsurpassed. After taking it in the form of hot tea, it takes thirty minutes for its active ingredients to enter the circulation; after one hour their concentration reaches its peak, then it begins to drop.

In the presence of an acute clinical condition or the first symptoms of a cold or flu, drink fresh juice tea every two or three hours so that the concentration of the active compounds in the bloodstream remains constant.

Fresh Ginger Juice Tea

Extract the juice from one or more pieces of ginger root. In total - for orientation - use an amount equal to that of a medium-large carrot, or four pieces the size of your thumb. Keep the leftover pulp from the juice extraction (you'll need it to make an infusion) or squeeze it out as much as you can to extract the juice to the last drop - there's always plenty left.

Pour 60 ml of fresh juice into a glass and a half of boiling water, add 1 tablespoon of wildflower honey, a quarter of squeezed lime and a pinch of cayenne pepper. Drink 4 to 6 cups per day.

Ginger infusion

Method 1. Infuse the part of the root left over from the juice extraction into one or two glasses of boiling water, depending on how much is left over, and leave the covered infusion to rest for 4-8 hours. Strain it and use it instead of the fresh juice to make the fresh juice tea described above. It will not be as effective as the freshly extracted juice, but almost.

Method 2. This is the method to use if you do not have an extractor or centrifuge to extract the juice from the ginger root. Grate the rhizome or chop it up as finely as possible - in this case just one piece, the size of your thumb. Put the mush in a container, cover it with a glass, a glass and a half of boiling water and let the infusion rest for 2-3 hours, covered, so that the essential oils do not disperse. Drink 4 to 6 glasses a day. In the acute phase of an illness. Drink at least 6 glasses per day of infusion.

The properties of ginger

As an antiviral, ginger has the following properties:

- Analgesic
- Anthelmintic

- Antiarthritic
- Antibacterial
- Antidiarroic
- Antiemetic
- Antifungal
- Anti-inflammatory
- Antispasmodic
- Anti-cough
- Carminative
- Blood circulation stimulant
- Diaphoretic
- Elastase inhibitor
- Hypotensive
- Immunostimulant
- Synergeist

Ginger is used mainly for these properties: it is a specific antiviral for respiratory diseases, a circulation stimulant that can also soothe nausea, diarrhea and abdominal cramps, lower fever (promoting sweating) and contain chills, reduce inflammation of the bronchi, dissolve phlegm, help expel it and improve coughing.

Used at the first symptoms of a cold or flu, and by this we mean the first day you have the feeling it is coming, it can reduce the course up to three days or even less, very often with a fairly mild symptomatology. When caught in the middle of a flu or cold episode, it helps to considerably improve the symptoms and accelerate healing.

Side effects and contraindications

Ginger is an emmenagogue, so during pregnancy high doses should be avoided; however, the dried root, in moderate doses, can help to alleviate pregnancy nausea. It can aggravate gallstones, so use it with caution. It can rarely promote abdominal distension, meteorism, stomach acidity and nausea (problems most often associated with the use of dried root powder).

Thyme and Plantain

Both thyme and plantain have distinct expectorant properties. This means that it promotes the removal of mucus from the trachea and bronchi, freeing the airways and improving the well-being of patients suffering from bronchial catarrh, chronic bronchitis, cough, sinusitis, colds, pneumonia, or other catarrhal diseases.

Both plants should be taken in the form of herbal tea, 3 to 4 cups per day. You can choose only one herb or combine them together.

The herbal tea is prepared by adding a teaspoon of dried (or freshly picked) grass to a cup of water. It is infused for 8-10 minutes and then filtered. It is important to drink the herbal tea while it is hot.

Lemon

Lemon can also help us fight viruses and is a natural remedy for colds and coughs. Try, for example, to take a glass of lukewarm water and lemon every morning when you wake up, still fasting: if taken constantly, this quick natural remedy will help to strengthen your immune system, as well as promote digestion. If you are looking for an even stronger remedy, try combining lemon and ginger: after boiling 1 litre of water, add the grated ginger root and wait for the liquid to boil; then cover the pot and wait 10 minutes. Finally, add the juice of 2 lemons. Drink hot or cold depending on your taste.

Ravinsara

In addition to having excellent antiviral qualities, Ravinsara also has anti-allergic and anti-inflammatory properties. Very effective against flu and colds, we can say that it is the most useful essential oil to face these problems since it is able to activate the immune system so that the response to external aggression is more effective and faster. Excellent to use also in prevention or to avoid contagion if there are already people at home with flu. For this purpose, of course, the best method is diffusion, which will help to purify the air in the rooms where you live.

Antiviral Essential Oils

Basil Essential Oil

Basil is anti-infective and antibacterial, which makes it an excellent choice. It can be used topically (with or without dilution, depending on skin sensitivity) and can also be used in cooking or taken internally via capsules to fight systemic infections.

Cassia essential oil

Other properties of cassia, besides antiviral, are antibacterial and antifungal. It must be diluted (1 drop of cassia to 4 drops of vector oil) and should not be taken internally but can be massaged in the reflex points or more areas of interest.

Cinnamon essential oil

Cinnamon has many properties, including antibacterial, anti-infective (especially urinary tract and intestinal tract), antiseptic and many others. It is strong, you must be sure to dilute it (1 drop of cinnamon and 3 drops of vector) but you can cook, bake or even prepare sweets to cure colds and flu.

Clove essential oil

This powerful oil is one of the best anti-viral essential oils, has strong antiseptic properties, and is also an excellent antifungal oil. Excellent for cleaning and diffusion, it is also antibacterial, disinfectant and antitumor. It can be used topically, diluted equally with a carrier oil, or taken internally with the right precautions. (consult your doctor).

Eucalyptus essential oil

Eucalyptus is a natural insecticide, antibacterial and anti-inflammatory which can usually be applied without dilution. Very useful for coughs and respiratory infections and gives great relief when massaged on the chest and throat.

Because of its effectiveness in the treatment of respiratory diseases, scientists have suggested that eucalyptus oil can be used as an alternative to medication to facilitate breathing. If you have a stuffy nose, pour a few drops of eucalyptus oil on a tissue and breathe deeply to relieve congestion of the nose, chest or upper chest.

Helichrysum essential oil

This interesting little oil is potently antiviral, but also antibacterial, antispasmodic and more. Excellent for healing, it can be used without dilution for most people, and is generally recognized as safe to consume.

Tea Tree Oil

Tea Tree oil is a powerful antiviral and antibacterial essential oil that is perfect for fighting the flu and cold virus. Tea tree oil is a well-researched essential oil that has many healing properties. For example, research published in the journal Antiviral Research found that tea tree oil can help fight the flu virus. In fact, other scientists have even stated that tea tree oil can almost be considered as a drug for various strains of influenza virus infections. The oil can be added to an inhaler or vapor diffuser to help eliminate germs in the air. Also, inhalation of tea tree oil in a steam bath reduces coughing, soothes sore throats and acts as a decongestant to eliminate mucus. You can also use a tea tree oil spray to disinfect surfaces to prevent the spread of influenza viruses.

Lemon essential oil

Lemon oil is an antioxidant, antiseptic and antitumor! It is great for cleansing, can be taken internally (dissolved in water) or used locally, although sensitive skin may require dilution.

Lime essential oil

This citrus oil is among the antiviral essential oils, but it is also antibacterial, antiseptic and tonic, among other things. It can be used without dilution, depending on skin sensitivity and can be taken internally (as in tea or with water). Caution: it can cause sensitivity to the sun with topical use up to 12 hours before, so we recommend using it before bedtime.

Malaleuca Essential Oil

One of the best anti-viral essential oils, melaleuca is also known for its anti-mycotic, antibacterial, anti-infective, antiparasitic, antiviral properties and, in addition, it helps tissue regeneration and is neurotonic. Sensitive skin may require dilution and is also an excellent cleanser.

Incense essential oil

Incense essential oil is a healing oil that can get rid of congestion and free you from a respiratory viral infection more quickly. Incense oil is a natural disinfectant, antiviral and anti-inflammatory essential oil. However, there are many other benefits of using incense as a home remedy for colds and flu. The magazine BMC Complementary Alternative Medicine reports that the compounds in incense have an antiviral effect against the influenza virus. This means that inhalation can help get rid of a viral infection in the respiratory tract and paranasal ducts. A disinfectant spray can also be used as an antiseptic to disinfect surfaces. Other medical studies of its properties have found that it can help relieve sneezing and runny noses.

It has also been found that incense contains healing compounds like those found in many anti-inflammatory painkillers used for headaches and muscle pain.

Lemongrass Oil

Lemongrass oil is an essential oil widely used as an alternative medicine to help reduce inflammation, the effects of viral infections and treat digestive problems. The benefits of using lemongrass in home remedies for colds or flu have been reported in the Journal of Advanced Pharmaceutical Technology & Research. In the study, researchers found that compounds in citronella extracts possess powerful antioxidant and antimicrobial properties. They also act as anti-inflammatories in the respiratory and digestive tract. Among the properties of lemongrass is its ability to reduce nausea, soothe headaches in a natural way, lower body temperatures and relieve muscle cramps. Lemongrass can help treat colds and flu symptoms because it helps to relax the mind and gives you a better night's rest. Getting plenty of sleep and rest is essential to help your body fight off a viral infection.

Lemon balm essential oil

Lemon balm oil is antibacterial, antimicrobial, antihistamine and you can also add a drop of it to your tea or apply it to the skin or reflex areas of the area of interest.

Lavender oil

Lavender oil may help to treat many of the symptoms associated with colds or flu like congestion, headaches, muscle aches, coughs, and insomnia. When it comes to making your own home remedy for flu and cold symptoms, lavender is an excellent all-rounder. For example, the Indian Journal of Pharmaceutical Sciences found that lavender can effectively treat sore throats and asthma symptoms. It also has an antimicrobial effect that can prevent the worsening of flu or cold symptoms. In addition, the European Journal of Dentistry reported that lavender is an excellent natural remedy for relieving colds and flu symptoms. The researchers said lavender is "antiseptic and anti-inflammatory for colds, flu and sinusitis and throat infections. You can also use lavender as a muscle scrub to help reduce stress and tension in sore muscles and joints.

On Guard" essential oil

Mixture of wild orange, cloves, cinnamon, eucalyptus and rosemary, is an oil that cures many diseases, infections and much more. It contains 5 essential oils and is particularly suitable for curing colds and flu, as well as for cleaning.

Oregano essential oil

Oregano is very powerful and antifungal. It is also very strong, which means that it should never be applied without diluting it first. But you can use it for cooking and it's great with mushrooms.

Peppermint essential oil

Peppermint is not only tasty (you can add oil to tea or water), but it is also a panacea for the digestive system. Besides being one of the most antiviral essential oils, it is also antibacterial, antispasmodic, antiseptic, anti-inflammatory and much more. Usually you can apply it without diluting it, to inhale in case of nausea, or to take internally.

Purifying" essential oil

Mixture of essential oils is specially created to be the cleaning of the body, but also of the house. It contains 6 essential oils (lemongrass, rosemary, malaleuca, lavender and myrtle), many of which are antiviral, antibacterial and even energizing. Great to use when the whole house has a cold or flu, topically or otherwise.

Thyme essential oil

Thyme is highly antibacterial, but also antiviral, antimicrobial and antiseptic. Excellent defence against many problems, although it should always be diluted (1 drop of thyme in 4 drops vector oil). It can be used in cooking, as well as any other "spicy" oil.

Sandalwood oil

Sandalwood oil can help improve your mood while your body is fighting a cold or flu. Sandalwood essential oil also has a sedative effect that can help reduce persistent coughing and sneezing. A 2016 report on natural remedies for treating nasal and sinus infections found that sandalwood can help reduce cold and flu symptoms. Researchers reported that sandalwood can help a person relax and reduce feelings of anxiety. Sandalwood essential oil also reduces the amount of nasal mucosa and helps remove congested airways.

NOTES

Usually, home remedies are enough to relieve the symptoms of an early and mild cold or flu virus. The antiviral and antimicrobial effect of many essential oils will also help prevent a worsening of upper respiratory tract infection. However, you should always consult your doctor if your symptoms become more severe.

In particular, <u>consult your doctor</u> in the following circumstances for severe cold or flu symptoms: with high fever together with sore throat, persistent cough and chest congestion; if cold or flu symptoms last several days; with severe earache; with mucus or phlegm in the bronchi.

Medical Herbalism for Beginners

HOMEMADE ANTIVIRAL PRODUCTS

Many of you do not know how to prepare essential oils to fight viral infections and diseases. (see chapter 4)

Here are a few examples that can help.

Natural antiviral cream

To prepare with shea butter base, or even beeswax. Add a total of 2-3 drops per gram of cream to one or more favourite essential oils and apply as needed. Store in a non-plastic container.

Natural antiviral ointments

The best base to use for an ointment would be coconut oil. Mix 1-4 drops of one or more antiviral essential oils. The application may vary depending on the strength of your oil, from every 2 hours for 2-3 times a day. Store in a glass jar, or a small bottle.

Natural antiviral bath salts

If possible, use "Epsom" salt (the high percentage of magnesium is good for your immune system) or sea salt and mix 3-5 drops of essential oils for every 1/4 cup of salt. Mix well in a glass container and spread up to 3/4 cup for each bath. This remedy is ideal for colds and chest constipation because the steam will also help ease any congestion.

Natural antiviral cleaning products

If the family is sick or there is a virus around, cleaning the house with antiviral essential oils can help kill the pathogens, while improving the immune defences of the whole family.

Antiviral Recipes

Do you want to learn how to prepare a powerful antivirus remedy?

It is important to consider the nutritional needs of the immune system and that is why we describe some anti-virus remedies recipes.

Lemon, Ginger and Honey

The main feature of this remedy is the combination of three very healthy and useful ingredients to give our immune system all the nutrients it needs to stay strong and able to fight against any type of infection.

Ingredients

- 2 large lemons, with rind
- ½ ginger root
- 200 ml organic honey (8 tablespoons)

Preparation

Before starting, wash the lemons well using a solution of water and vinegar to disinfect them and remove any pesticide residues. It is also important to use the lemon peel as this is where many of the nutrients are concentrated, including a good dose of vitamin C.

Wash the ginger root well, cut it into small pieces and blend it with the sliced lemon. Add the honey last and blend all the ingredients well until you get a homogeneous mixture.

When your mixture is ready, pour it into an airtight glass container and keep it in the fridge.

If you keep this remedy in the refrigerator for a long time and notice that the honey begins to crystallize, a good solution is to heat it in a bain-marie so as not to waste it.

For those over 13 years of age, it is advisable to consume one spoonful a day.

The dose for children, on the other hand, is a maximum of one teaspoon per day. You can dissolve it in tea, water or other hot drinks.

Olive leaf infusion

Thanks to the oleuropein contained in them, olive leaves have excellent antibacterial, anti-inflammatory and antioxidant properties. They allow to eliminate bacteria, viruses and fungi, also stimulating the immune system. The active principles that characterize them also allow to keep diabetes at bay, decreasing blood sugar levels, to control hypertension and to provide a valuable aid in case of osteoporosis and arthritis. Olive leaves also have pain-relieving properties. They are also useful to mitigate skin damage caused by ultraviolet rays and free radicals.

The benefits are not over here. The leaves have anti-tumor properties and prevent Alzheimer's disease. The beneficial effects are manifold and can be obtained by drinking the infusion.

The infusion of olive leaves is remarkably beneficial for our health, performing many important actions. Here are all the benefits.

Antiviral, antibacterial, antifungal. It strengthens the immune system, helping to prevent various diseases. It counteracts herpes, flu and cold viruses.

Reduces fever. The infusion helps to lower body temperature.

Antitumoral and antiproliferative, especially in case of breast cancer and melanoma.

Antioxidant: slows cellular aging, counteracts free radicals.

Reduces blood pressure, promotes peripheral vasodilation.

Reduces blood glucose promotes the reduction of blood glucose levels. Keeps diabetes under control.

Reduces bad cholesterol, increases good cholesterol.

Fights gout, arthritis and rheumatoid arthritis.

Painkiller. Reduces joint pain.

Prevents osteoporosis.

Prevents cardiovascular diseases has a powerful antithrombotic action.

Reduces hemorrhoids and hematomas: it strengthens the capillary walls, reducing the bleeding symptoms of hemorrhoids.

Prevents Alzheimer's: it is neuroprotective.

Reduces reflux and gastritis: it has an antacid effect. This characteristic has not been discovered as a result of scientific studies but is based on the experience of some people suffering from gastritis, who have stated that they feel better when taking one or two teaspoons of olive leaf infusion after meals.

It fights chronic fatigue.

Slimming effect: helps to lose weight and burn excess abdominal fat.

More than an infusion, we should talk about decoction. To prepare it, it is advisable to use leaves from organic cultivation. This is how it is prepared.

Put 10 grams of fresh olive leaves or 5 grams of dried leaves in a pot with 250 ml of cold water.

Bring to the boil. When the water starts to boil, lower the heat and leave to cook for 15 minutes.

Filter the infusion and let it cool slightly. Now you can drink it.

How to take it

The infusion should simply be drunk in order to get all the benefits it can offer. You can drink one to three cups a day. If the taste is too bitter for your palate, you can make it more pleasant and sweet by adding a little honey.

You can prepare a larger amount of infusion and store it in the refrigerator in a bottle. For 1 litre of decoction you need 40 grams of fresh leaves or 20 grams of dried leaves.

Contraindications and side effects

The decoction of olive leaves is not recommended for those taking drugs with hypotensive action, especially if they are vasodilator drugs. This is because the infusion could increase their action.

Side effects include allergic skin reactions, sometimes accompanied by allergic asthma for those who suffer from allergies caused by olive tree derivatives and other plants belonging to the Oleaceae family.

Before taking the infusion, it is always advisable to consult your doctor, especially if you are taking medication.

Echinacea infusions

Echinacea herbal tea is obtained from the dried and chopped plant and from its root, which is then placed inside sachets or sold loose for the preparation of the herbal tea. It is not possible to quantify and standardise the percentage of active substances in the preparation of the herbal tea and therefore it may not be very concentrated or too concentrated. However, it is recommended to use a maximum of 2 cups of decoction per day for a maximum of 2 consecutive weeks. The echinacea decoction is prepared by adding one tablespoon of dried root echinacea to 200 ml of cold water. This is brought to the boil and kept for 5 minutes, then it is removed from the heat and left to rest in infusion for another 10 minutes. It is filtered and drunk by adding honey, lemon juice or other natural sweeteners to taste.

Decoction for external and internal use

Echinacea decoction is useful both for external use for wraps and washing on skin that has scars, dermatitis, irritation, inflammation, canker sores or other skin problems. It brings with it immunostimulant, anti-inflammatory, protective, healing properties, thus creating a suitable environment that accelerates the regeneration of epithelial tissues and soothes infections. In addition, this echinacea decoction is used for all the problems we have previously indicated and for coughs, colds, sore throats and flu.

Recipe with echinacea and rose hips

With the same preparation of the echinacea decoction we can make it and add half a tablespoon of cinorrodi berries, i.e. rosehips. Remember to leave the decoction to rest for at least 10 minutes to allow all the active ingredients to come out of the herbs and be poured into the herbal tea. These two medicinal plants are enhanced because the properties of echinacea are added to the properties of rose hips, very rich in vitamin C, helps to strengthen the immune system, fight infections and relieve respiratory diseases.

Recipe with echinacea and marshmallow roots

Another formulation is the decoction of echinacea roots and marshmallow roots. The preparation remains the same as the decoction with a level spoon of echinacea and a level spoon of marshmallow. This decoction can be used externally with wraps and washes to help the healing and regeneration of the epidermis when there are skin problems. Thanks to the presence of its mucilage, marshmallow adds emollient, soothing and flaming properties to those of echinacea. Besides its external use, drinking the decoction of echinacea and marshmallow also helps the mucous membranes of the gastrointestinal tract and strengthens the immune system.

Suffumigias with essential oil

To quickly clear the obstructed airways, bring a pot of water to the boil, remove it from the fire, bend your head over the pot and cover the back of your neck with a towel, creating a sort of "curtain" around the pot, and breathe deeply with your nose for 30 seconds.

To increase the decongestant effect, add one or two drops of mint or eucalyptus essential oil to the water.

Licorice herbal tea

You need about 60 grams of dry root per 1 litre of water or 2 or 3 pieces for a single cup of water. These need to boil for a long time (about an hour) in order to release all their active ingredients.

Mint herbal tea

Refreshing and purifying mint is perfect especially in summer! The herbal tea obtained from the leaves of this plant can be prepared in advance and stored in the refrigerator to consume it when needed. To make it even tastier you can also add a few slices of lemon.

Curcuma herbal tea

There are several variants of curcuma herbal tea, all perfect to prepare in advance so that they can be cooled and consumed throughout the day. Thanks to the presence of the "queen of spices", this drink is enriched with many beneficial properties: it purifies the body acting on the liver, promotes digestion, increases the immune defences, improves circulation and is anti-inflammatory.

Curcuma herbal tea is a very easy drink to prepare to fully enjoy the benefits of this spice with a thousand properties. It can be prepared from powdered or fresh curcuma and flavoured at will.

If you want to take curcuma herbal tea for healing purposes, contact your trusted herbalist to find out the best doses and methods of preparation according to your health condition.

Preparing curcuma herbal tea is very simple and you can start with either fresh curcuma or powdered curcuma, depending on what is indicated in the different recipes below.

Don't forget that curcuma can also have contraindications, for example for those who suffer from gallstones, so if you have any doubts, consult your doctor, even about natural remedies.

Curcuma herbal tea powder

With curcuma powder you can prepare an herbal tea useful especially in case of cold and sore throat.

- 500 ml of water
- 2 teaspoons of curcuma powder
- 1 teaspoon of honey
- 1 tablespoon of lemon juice
- 1 pinch of black pepper

In 500 millilitres of hot water dissolve 2 teaspoons of curcuma powder and add 1 teaspoon of honey, a tablespoon of lemon juice and a pinch of black pepper. Mix carefully and drink one or two cups of curcuma tea a day. The black pepper is used to help the absorption of curcuma in our body.

Fresh curcuma herbal tea

- 250 ml of water
- 5 grams of fresh grated curcuma

The herbal tea with fresh curcuma is prepared in the form of a decoction. Bring the water together with the freshly grated curcuma to the boil in a saucepan and let it simmer for 5 minutes. Then let it cool down, sweeten with honey or malt if you want and drink your herbal tea in the morning on an empty stomach or after meals to aid digestion. You can add a pinch of black pepper.

Curcuma and Ginger Herbal Tea

- 500 ml of water
- 2 slices of fresh ginger
- 2 teaspoons of fresh grated curcuma
- 2 slices of lemon
- 2 teaspoons of honey or malt

Grate the fresh curcuma and break up the ginger. Bring them to the boil in a saucepan together with water and slices of lemon, to choose organic and untreated. Let it simmer for about 10 minutes, then filter and drink sweetening to taste.

Curcuma herbal tea and matcha tea

- 250 ml of water
- 1 teaspoon of curcuma
- ½ teaspoon matcha
- ½ teaspoon of cinnamon
- 1 pinch of nutmeg
- 1 pinch of vanilla berry powder

Curcuma herbal tea is matcha tea is energizing mainly because of this precious stimulating tea. Pour the water and all the ingredients into a pot. Heat up by stirring until the tea is almost boiling. If needed, stir with a fork or a small whisk, or with the matcha tea whisk. Then pour into the cups and if you want add honey and lemon juice.

Curcuma and spice tea

- 250 ml of water
- 1 teaspoon of curcuma powder
- 1 pinch of cinnamon
- 1 pinch of powdered cloves
- 1 pinch of nutmeg
- 1 pinch of black pepper
- 2 tablespoons of almond milk or coconut milk
- 1 teaspoon of honey

Heat and simmer in a saucepan for 10 minutes all the ingredients except almond milk (or other vegetable milk) and honey. Then pour everything into a cup and season to taste with honey and almond milk or your favourite vegetable milk.

Curcuma lemonade

It's delicious and will make you feel better in the long run. What it takes to make curcuma lemonade:

- 5 cups of water
- 4 tablespoons of freshly grated curcuma root

- 3 tablespoons of raw honey
- 2 teaspoons of grated ginger
- ½ cup fresh lemon juice
- ½ cup orange juice (optional for taste)

Preparation

Boil the 5 cups of water and place the grated curcuma and ginger in a container that can hold hot water. Then pour the boiled water into the container. Let the mixture rest for at least 10 minutes, then add the honey that you will stir until it melts completely.

Filter the mixture and add lemon juice and, if you like, orange juice. After it has cooled a bit, sip it and you will feel better!

Thyme herbal tea

Preparing thyme herbal tea is very simple, in fact it is only necessary:

- 1 handful of dried thyme
- 250 ml of water

Boil the water, then add thyme and let it boil for a minute, turn off the heat and let it cool before filtering and drinking. Since thyme is not everyone's taste, you can add a teaspoon of honey or another natural sweetener of your choice.

It is recommended to drink it on an empty stomach, for example, in the evening before going to sleep. The benefits will begin to be felt after a few days of intake.

Eucalyptus and sage herbal tea

Eucalyptus herbal tea clears the respiratory tract and is useful in case of colds. Eucalyptus can be combined with other useful herbs in this case, such as sage. Pour one teaspoon of dried sage and one teaspoon of dried eucalyptus into a cup of boiling water, leave to rest for up to 10 minutes, filter and drink. Sage herbal tea is contraindicated during pregnancy and breastfeeding, in case of hypertension and epilepsy.

Lemon balm herbal tea

Lemon balm is a plant with excellent calming and sedative properties, useful in case of colds. It stimulates sweating, an important aspect that can help lower the fever and eliminate toxins trapped in the body. To prepare an herbal tea, pour 1 teaspoon of dried lemon balm into each cup of boiling water, leave to rest 5 minutes and filter. Find the lemon balm loose or in sachets in an herbalist's shop. Lemon balm is easy to grow in pots or in the garden, so you can pick the leaves and dry them to use when you need them.

Cinnamon herbal tea

Cinnamon tea is excellent for reducing inflammation of the throat and against winter sickness. Bring to the boil the amount of water contained in a normal cup together with 2 teaspoons of honey, 2 or 3 teaspoons of cinnamon powder and 1 pinch of pepper. Drinking it still warm will have a magical effect on the respiratory tract.

Golden milk

It is a curcuma-based drink with numerous benefits, which is recommended especially for those suffering from joint problems and those seeking a natural anti-inflammatory.

Ingredients:

- Half cup of water (120 ml)
- 60 gr curcuma
- rice milk
- sweet almond oil for food use
- 1 tablespoon of honey
- Cinnamon

Put the water in a saucepan and add the curcuma.

Cook until all the water is dry. Stir to prevent lumps from forming.

At the end, you'll get a curcuma cream. Pour the mixture into a glass container, cover with a plate and put in the fridge.

This amount will be enough for about 40 days.

Pour the rice milk into a small pot and heat. Add a teaspoon of the curcuma mixture and dissolve it in the milk.

Pour into a cup and add a teaspoon of sweet almond oil for food use, a teaspoon of honey and a sprinkle of cinnamon.

Now you can drink your Golden Milk.

ANTIVIRAL GASTRONOMY

The change of season, as every year, has brought the flu, forcing us to spend the canons four days under the covers waiting for the congestion to pass. But to fight it and prevent it, we can start from the table, choosing to fill up with: vitamin C (contained in citrus fruits, helps prevent colds), allicin (present in garlic, has antibiotic and antiviral properties), flavonoids (present in onions, fight bacteria and work in synergy with vitamin C) and ginger, precious to fight fever and cough.

28 Recipes to Fight Flu with Natural Methods

Fish Dishes

Cod terrine with ginger and lime sauce

Duration: 3 h Level: Easy Doses: 4 people

Ingredients:

- 500 g cod fillets
- 70 g cottage cheese
- 2 spring onions
- 2 egg whites

- 1 lime
- 1 lemon
- Milk
- Butter
- Shallot
- Mustard
- fresh ginger
- chives
- mint and parsley
- extra virgin olive oil
- salt and black pepper grains
- salad for garnish

For the cod terrine recipe, put the fish in a saucepan, cover it flush with cold water, add a pinch of salt, ground pepper, a few sprigs of parsley, a quarter of shallot, half a lemon and cook for 10'. Drain the fish and blend it with the egg whites, the ricotta, a tablespoon of milk, the juice of half a lemon, the grated rind, a few strands of chives and a few chopped leaves of parsley and mint. Butter a rectangular mould (28×8 cm, h 7 cm), line it with baking paper, butter it too, then pour the fish mixture.

Level it with a spatula, cover it with aluminium foil and bake it in a bain-marie at 180 °C and cook it for 30 minutes. Take the bowl out of the oven, let it cool, then put it in the fridge for at least 2 hours. Prepare the accompanying sauce by blending 40 g of oil with the juice of half a lime, a teaspoon of mustard, a teaspoon of grated ginger, salt and pepper.

Divide the spring onions in half along the length and fry them in a pan with a drizzle of oil. Slice the bowl into large slices and garnish them with the stewed onions, a few leaves of salad, a little grated lemon zest.

Roasted mackerel with mashed orange and carrots

Duration: 1 h 10 min Level: Medium Doses: 6 people

Ingredients:

- 3 mackerels
- 400 g potatoes
- 50 g rice milk
- 50 g carrot
- 30 g orange juice
- 20 g orange peel
- 10 g prune
- balsamic vinegar
- sugar
- orange
- extra virgin olive oil
- salt and white pepper

Fillet the mackerel, sprinkle them with salt, white pepper and sugar, let them marinate for 15', then rinse them, dry them with kitchen paper, check that there are no bones and, if necessary, remove them with tweezers. Also remove the transparent film covering the side of the skin.

Wash the potatoes well and collect them in an ovenproof dish, seal it with the film suitable for cooking in the microwave. Bake them in the microwave and cook them for 7-9 minutes, depending on the size of the potatoes; let them cool down, then peel them and mash them; add 40 g of oil stirring with a whisk, lukewarm rice milk a little at a time, orange juice, salt and the grated rind of an orange.

Cut the carrot into slices about 3 mm thick, dip them in boiling water for 1', cool them and season with balsamic vinegar. Cut the prune into small pieces. Peel 2 slices of orange and cut them into chunks. Boil the orange peels 3 times in water, each time new. Then blend them together with 45 g of water, a pinch of salt and one of sugar.

Cook the mackerel for 20 seconds per side in a hot non-stick pan with a drizzle of oil, let it rest in the pan for a few minutes. Spread a strip of mash on the plate, sit on top of the mackerel, on the side the carrot slices and the prune, complete with the orange peel sauce and a few pieces of peeled orange.

Scallops with orange and avocado sauce

Duration: 2 h 30 min Level: Medium Doses: 6 people

Ingredients:

- 180 g mature avocado
- 6 scallops
- Parsley
- Shallot
- Orange and lemon
- red radicchio
- extra virgin olive oil
- salt and pepper

Remove the corals from the scallops and cut the walnuts into slices; beat them lightly with a meat tenderizer between two sheets of baking paper. Dress them with lemon juice and salt and let them marinate for 2 hours covered in the fridge.

Mash the peeled avocado with a drop of lemon, salt, pepper, a tuft of chopped parsley, 3 washers of chopped shallot and a drizzle of oil.

Spread the sauce in the shells, add the radicchio fillets, the marinated scallops and complete with peeled orange cubes.

Broccoli and clams' soup with orange passatelli

Duration: 1 h Level: Easy Doses: 6 people

Ingredients:

- 1 Kg purged clams
- 500 g broccoli
- 220 g wholemeal breadcrumbs
- 120 g grated Parmesan cheese
- 100 g oatmeal
- 5 eggs
- Orange
- Garlic and parsley
- extra virgin olive oil
- salt

For the recipe of broccoli and clam soup with orange passatelli, mix the breadcrumbs with the parmesan cheese, oatmeal, eggs, a pinch of salt and the grated rind of a small orange. Form a dough ball, put it in a bowl, seal it with film and let it rest in the fridge for 30 minutes. Blanch the broccoli tops and drain them al dente.

Brown half of the broccoli tops in a pan with a drizzle of oil and a clove of chopped garlic; add the clams, cover them and let them open. Remove the clams and shell them. Finely blend the broccoli and cooking liquid with a tuft of chopped parsley. Prepare the passatelli with the appropriate tool (you can also use the potato masher with the disc with the larger holes). Boil them for 5' in boiling salted water, then drain them in a pan with the broccoli shake, the remaining tops, the shelled clams and after a few minutes turn off.

Distribute them on the plates. Complete with a drizzle of raw oil and grated orange peel.

Scampi, ginger and rhubarb.

Duration: 1 h Level: Medium Doses: 4 people

Ingredients:

- 180 g rhubarb
- 30 g fresh ginger
- 20 whole scampi
- celery stalks
- onion
- extra virgin olive oil
- salt

For the scampi recipe, ginger and rhubarb in broth, remove the scampi from the head with the claws; cut the heads in half and rinse them by removing the entrails, then dip them in 2 litres of unsalted water scented with half a peeled onion and 2 celery stalks and cook the broth for 30 minutes from boiling. Wash and chop the rhubarb.

Thread the tails of the scampi, with the shell, on wooden skewers, making sure that they remain well stretched. Filter the broth and pour it into a large saucepan; add salt, add the peeled and thinly sliced ginger and bring back to the boil; then add the scampi skewers and the rhubarb in chunks and cook them for 5 minutes.

Drain the scampi skewers, ginger and rhubarb from the soup. Filter the broth; peel the scampi and remove the skewers. Serve the soup with the scampi, rhubarb and ginger, and top it off with a drizzle of oil.

Scampi with ginger and fennel

Duration: 40 min Level: Easy Doses: 4 people

Ingredients:

- 40 g raisins
- 20 g fresh peeled ginger
- 16 shelled langoustine tails
- 2 very firm mandarins
- a fennel
- sage
- extra virgin olive oil
- salt and pepper

For the recipe of scampi browned with ginger and fennel, soak the raisins. Arrange the langoustine tails on a plate and perfume them with the grated rind of a mandarin, salt and pepper. Let them rest in the fridge covered with film for about ten minutes. Peel the fennel and cut it into not too thin slices.

Cut the ginger into small pieces, brown them in a pan with 2 tablespoons of oil for 1-2', then add the fennel slices and continue for 2', wet with a ladleful of hot water, add the squeezed raisins and complete the cooking in another 10'. Collect in a pan 2 tablespoons of oil, 3-4 tangerine peel and 2 sage leaves; heat and then blanch the scampi on a high flame for a couple of minutes.

Spread the fennel slices, raisins, ginger chunks, scampi and complete with sage leaves browned in a veil of oil.

Bruschetta with thyme and lemon with scampi

Duration: 30 min Level: Easy Doses: 4 people

Ingredients:

- 8 pcs Slices of homemade bread
- 3 pcs Spring onions
- 8 pcs Shelled Norway lobster tails
- 1 pcs Ripe Tomato
- 1 pcs Thyme bunch
- Acacia honey
- Lemon

- Extra virgin olive oil
- salt

Line a baking paper plate, place the slices of bread in the oven and bake them at 170 °C for 5'.

Flip a bunch of thyme.

Peel the spring onions, preserving some green and slice them into slices of salami.

Brown them in a little oil for 1', then reduce the heat, add a teaspoon of thyme leaves, a grated lemon rind, a teaspoon of honey and continue cooking for 2-3'.

Cut the tomato into four slices.

Rub the slices of bread taken out of the oven with the slices of ripe tomato, salt them and season them with a grated lemon rind and the rest of the thyme.

Heat a frying pan veiled with oil; when it is hot, burn the langoustine tails shelled for 1' on one side only. Salt.

Spread the onions on the slices of bread, complete with the scampi and serve immediately.

Sole fillets with grapefruit.

Duration: 1 h 30 min Level: Medium Doses: 4 people

Ingredients:

- 4 medium soles
- 2 onions

- 1 grapefruit
- 1 pink grapefruit
- celery stalks
- flour
- butter
- sugar
- salt

For the recipe of sole fillets with grapefruit, peel and fillet the sole, remove the entrails and heads. Prepare a broth with the bones: cook them in a litre of water with a peeled onion and a couple of celery stalks for 30'. Peel the pink grapefruit and cut it into slices; mix it in a bowl with a level spoon of sugar and a level teaspoon of salt; after 10', drain it, place it on a plate covered with baking paper and put it in the freezer for at least 1 hour.

Peel and chop 1/2 onion, let it wither in a saucepan with 40 g of butter for 5', then add the remaining grapefruit juice and reduce the liquid for 10', then add half a litre of filtered sole broth and cook for another 15'; finally blend and sieve everything through a fine strainer (if the sauce is too liquid, thicken it by adding a teaspoon of corn starch diluted in a cup of hot water).

Take the grapefruit out of the freezer, chop it with a knife and put it back in the freezer until it is ready to use. Flour the sole fillets and fry them in a knob of butter for 2-3 minutes on each side, salt and serve hot accompanied by the frosty grapefruit grains.

Agliata octopus

Duration: 1 h 10 min Level: Easy Doses: 6 people

Ingredients:

- 1 Kg octopus
- 200 g tomato puree
- 200 g vinegar
- 100 g dried tomatoes in oil
- 25 g capers in salt plus a little thyme
- Laurel
- Parsley and garlic
- extra virgin olive oil
- salt

For the garlic octopus recipe, eviscerate and wash the octopus then put it in a saucepan covered with cold water, with a sprig of thyme and a bay leaf. Bring it to the boil and cook it for 30 minutes, then let it cool in its water. Drain the octopus, remove the eyes and beak and cut it into chunks.

Chop the drained dried tomatoes and rinse the capers with salt. Chop them with a tuft of parsley and half a clove of garlic. Brown the chopped tomatoes in about 100 g of oil for 2-3', then add the vinegar and tomato puree and cook for another 15'; season with salt if necessary.

Add the chopped octopus to the sauce and let it flavour for 2', adding a pinch of chopped parsley and capers. Leave to cool, put in the fridge for at least 12 hours to rest.

Garlic cream and anchovy fillets

Duration: 1 h Level: Easy Doses: 4 people

Ingredients:

- 500 g potatoes
- 7 peeled garlic cloves
- 4 anchovy fillets in oil
- 2 slices of bread
- Shallot
- white wine
- vegetable stock
- extra virgin olive oil
- coarse and fine salt
- pepper

For the recipe of the garlic cream with crispy bread and anchovy fillets, pour in a saucepan a drizzle of extra virgin olive oil and a pinch of coarse salt, bring on the fire and brown half chopped shallot.

Add the peeled and chopped potatoes, 5 cloves of garlic, blend with a splash of white wine, then cover with 800 g of hot broth and cook for 40'. Turn off, remove the garlic cloves and blend the rest with the immersion blender to obtain a thick cream. Return it to the fire, season with salt and pepper.

Slice the remaining cloves of garlic into thin flakes and brown them in a pan with a drizzle of extra virgin olive oil. Release the pan and toast the slices of bread greased with extra virgin olive oil in the same pan. Distribute the garlic cream in bowls and complete it, before serving, with the roughly chopped slices of bread, the fried garlic and an anchovy fillet.

Bread with cuttlefish and ginger potatoes

Duration: 1 h 15 min Level: Medium Doses: 4 people

Ingredients:

- 350 g cuttlefish
- 4 potatoes
- 400 g asparagus
- 70 g fresh peeled ginger
- 24 slices of homemade bread
- Basil, garlic and extra virgin olive oil
- Salt and pepper

For the recipe of mille-feuille bread with cuttlefish and ginger potatoes, boil the potatoes with the peel for 30-40', depending on the size. Spread the slices of bread on a baking sheet lined with baking paper, cover them with another sheet of baking paper and place them on a second baking sheet: this way the slices will not curl during cooking. Bake at 120 °C for 10-15'.

Peel the asparagus, cut them into very thin ribbons and dress them with oil, salt and pepper. Blanch the cuttlefish sacks in unsalted boiling water for 1', drain them, cool them in cold water for less than 1', drain them and dry them quickly with kitchen paper.

Open the bags for a long time, to obtain a kind of triangle and then make some light cross engravings. Sauté them in a pan in a veil of oil with a clove of garlic and a sprig of basil for 2-3'. Cut the ginger and blend it with half a glass of water. Peel the potatoes, mash them in a potato masher, salt them, pepper them; mix them with 4 tablespoons of oil and 1-3 tablespoons of the blended ginger, dosing the quantity according to your taste. If you want to obtain a very fine cream, sieve it.

Spread the hot potato cream on a slice of bread passed in the oven, add a few strips of asparagus, then put another slice of bread, more potato cream and asparagus and close with another slice. Make the other 7 mille-feuilles in this way. Serve immediately two each with the hot cuttlefish, decorating with a few basil leaves.

Fish and onion hot dogs

Duration: 50 min Level: Medium Doses: 6 people

Ingredients:

- 300 g clean cuttlefish
- 300 g onions
- 200 g fillets of sea bass
- 180 g fresh cream
- 6 hot dog sandwiches
- 5 egg whites
- mustard grains
- pickled cucumbers
- extra virgin olive oil
- salt

Peel the fillets of sea bass and remove the bones; rinse the cuttlefish; blend them together, then add the egg whites, a good pinch of salt and blend again, obtaining a homogeneous mixture. Transfer it into a bowl, place it on top of a container full of water and ice (this step is used to thicken the mixture in the next step); now add the cream and stir.

Divide the mixture into 6 equal portions, transfer them onto 6 sheets of film and shape them into narrow, long strands. Wrap them in the film (choose the type suitable for cooking), obtaining similar rolls in the shape of sausages (ø 3 cm, length 20 cm); close the ends with string and boil them in a large pot of boiling water, slightly salted, for about ten minutes.

Peel the onions and slice them thinly, then brown them in a veil of oil with a pinch of salt for about ten minutes, until they appear golden. Finely slice 5-6 gherkins. Drain the rolls and gently remove them from the film. Cut the sandwiches and prepare 6 hot dogs: spread a spoonful of mustard on the base, arrange a few slices of gherkin, onions, finally the fish sausage and close with a sandwich.

Meat Dishes

Garganelli with agretti, ginger and lamb sauce

Duration: 2 h Level: Medium Doses: 4 people

Ingredients:

- 400 g lamb shoulder meat
- 200 g flour
- 120 g hulled agretti

- 100 g durum wheat semolina
- 30 g fresh ginger
- 3 yolks
- 2 eggs
- 2 celery stalks
- 1 sachet of saffron
- 1 shallot
- grated Parmesan cheese
- curcuma powder
- thyme
- dry white wine
- extra virgin olive oil
- salt and pepper

Preparation

For the garganelli recipe with agretti, ginger and lamb ragout, mix the flour and semolina with the eggs, yolks, saffron and a tablespoon of curcuma. You will have to obtain a firm dough; if it is difficult to work, add a little water. Wrap the dough in the film and let it rest for 1 hour. Reduce the lamb flesh into small cubes. Cut the celery into cubes and chop the shallot. Brown the lamb flesh in a saucepan with the celery, shallot, 2 tablespoons of oil and a teaspoon of chopped thyme; after 1-2' wet with a glass of white wine, let the alcohol evaporate, cover with water and continue to cook for 1 hour. At the end, salt and pepper. Blanch the agretti for less than 1'. Drain them. Peel the ginger, grate it and squeeze the pulp for juice. Saute the agretti in a pan with the ginger juice, 2 tablespoons of oil and the lamb sauce for a couple of minutes.

Roll out the pasta into a very thin sheet and cut it into squares about 4-5 cm wide. Place a stick on the corner of a square and roll up the square then pull out the stick to obtain a "garganello". Repeat these operations with all the other squares. Boil the "garganelli" in boiling salted water for 2-3 minutes and drain them in the pan, stir well, remove from heat, stir with 1-2 tablespoons of grain and serve immediately.

Terrine of hare and caramelized onions

Duration: 4 h Level: Medium Doses: 6 people

Ingredients:

- 500 g hare thighs or shoulders
- 260 g red onions
- 200 g cold butter
- 150 g wine vinegar
- 100 g fresh cream
- 100 g sugar
- 30 g leek with washers
- fennel beards

- homemade bread
- garlic
- extra virgin olive oil
- Salt and pepper grains

Dip the hare legs in a saucepan full of salted water with 2 peppercorns, a clove of garlic with the peel. Since it comes to the boil, cook over the heat for at least 50'. Let the hare legs cool in the cooking stock, then peel them and filter the stock. Melt a knob of butter in a frying pan, add the leek and hare flesh, salt, pepper and cream and cook everything for 10-12 minutes on a high flame. Turn off and whisk in cream in the food processor with a ladle of filtered broth.

When the mixture is homogeneous enough, add 200 g of cold butter in tufts, continuing to blend. Blend until a fine grain is obtained. Distribute the hare terrine in one or more small bowls, seal them with the film and let them cool in the fridge for at least 2 hours. Collect the vinegar, sugar, a tablespoon of oil and sliced onions in a saucepan and stew them gently for 20-22 minutes.

Slice the bread and toast it in a pan or in the oven for 2-3'. Serve the hare terrine on the toasted bread and top with the caramelized onions and fennel beets.

Ginger veal beating with ginger

Duration: 20 min Level: Easy Doses: 8 people

Ingredients:

- 400 g veal fillet
- 180 g fennel
- 80 g carrots
- 3 radishes
- fresh ginger
- lemon
- extra virgin olive oil
- salt

For the recipe for the ginger veal fillet, finely chop the veal fillet with a knife until you get a beat. Slice the carrots and fennel into slices, keeping some green beards aside.

Peel the radishes and cut them into 8 slices. Peel a small piece of ginger and chop it very finely; put it in a bowl with 4 tablespoons of oil, the juice of half a lemon, a pinch of salt and the chopped green fennel: mix to obtain a vinaigrette.

Season the meat and vegetables with the vinaigrette and serve immediately.

Crushed chicken and baked garlic

Duration: 1 h 20 min Level: Easy Doses: 4 people

Medical Herbalism for Beginners

Ingredients:

- 1 pcs Cleaned and gutted chicken
- 4 pcs Garlic heads
- Thyme
- Butter
- Rosemary
- Tomato Concentrate
- Mint, Sage and Garlic
- White wine vinegar
- Extra virgin olive oil
- Salt and Pepper

Make two clean cuts in the back of the chicken along the entire spine so that it is completely removed, then open the chicken by squeezing it with energy.

Blend 5-6 sage leaves, the leaves of a few tufts of rosemary, the leaves of 3 sprigs of thyme and 4-5 leaves of mint, a tablespoon of tomato paste, a tablespoon of white wine vinegar,
a clove of peeled garlic and a tablespoon of water.
Spread the aromatic mixture on the crushed chicken, salt and pepper.
Heat a large saucepan veiled with oil that can go in the oven and cook the chicken on the side of the flesh for 5 minutes on a high flame.

Remove from the heat and gently insert butter flakes between the skin and the flesh of the chicken.

Peel the garlic heads, remove only the outer sheath, taking care not to separate the cloves, grease them with oil, salt and pepper and place them in the saucepan with the chicken.

Bake at 200 °C for 50'.

Take the chicken out of the oven and serve it immediately with the garlic heads on the side.

Vegetable Dishes

Carrot gazpacho with celeriac

Duration: 1 h 20 min Level: Easy Doses: 4 people

Ingredients:

- 650 g Carrots
- 600 g Celeriac
- 250 g Orange juice
- 70 g Celery leaves
- 40 g Hazelnuts
- 2 Celery stems
- Sliced rye bread
- Lemon juice
- sweet curry
- Brown sugar

- Extra virgin olive oil
- Salt and Pink Pepper

Peel the celeriac, grate it with the grater with large holes and then stew it in a casserole with oil and salt for about 45 minutes. Peel the carrots and cut them into chunks. Cut the celery stalks into very thin fillets and soak them in cold water so that they become crispy. Collect the carrots in a saucepan with 20 g of oil, salt and a teaspoon of curry; bring to the heat with the lid and cook gently for 30 minutes, stirring occasionally. Turn them off and let them cool.

Blend the carrots with the orange juice, 4 tablespoons of lemon juice, 15 g of brown sugar, 30g of oil and 30g of water. You will obtain a very smooth cream (gazpacho). Wash the celery leaves, boil them for 1', drain them, cool them and blend them with 100 g of oil and a tablespoon of celeriac stew.

Blend the hazelnuts with 40 g of oil and 30 g of water. Then add the celeriac. Spread the celeriac and hazelnut puree on the slices of rye bread, season with celery leaf sauce, a few grains of crushed pink pepper, complete with the crispy celery fillets drained and serve with gazpacho.

Crushed Onions

Duration: 2 h 30 min

Level: Easy

Doses: 4 people

Ingredients:

- 500 g Onions
- 400 g Flour
- 40 g Lard (or extra virgin olive oil)
- 10 g Fresh brewer's yeast
- Extra virgin olive oil
- Sugar and Salt

Knead the flour, lard, yeast and a teaspoon of sugar with 220 g of lukewarm water; when the ingredients start to be mixed, add 10 g of salt and knead the mixture until a smooth dough is obtained. Leave it to rise covered for about 1 hour, until the volume doubles.

Then crush the dough in the oven tray greased with oil (or in two round trays, ø 24 cm) and let it rest for another 20-30 minutes. Peel the onions and cut them into slices; blanch them in boiling water for 5 minutes, drain them well and place them on top of the buns. Season with oil and salt and bake at 200 °C for 25-30 minutes.

Onion Soup

Duration: 1 h Level: Easy Doses: 4 people

Ingredients:

- 1 Kg white onions
- 300 g vegetable stock
- 200 g slices of wholemeal bread
- 120 g fontina
- 50 g butter
- salt

Peel the onions and slice them very thinly. Brown them in a pan with butter for 7-8'. Season with salt and cook them stirring often for another 20 minutes.

Place a layer of wholemeal bread in an ovenproof dish, cover it with onions, then make another layer of bread and onions. Cover the surface with filleted grated fontina cheese and wet everything with the broth.

Bake the baking dish at 200 °C for about 15 minutes. Remove from the oven and serve hot.

Fennel with Catalan sauce

Duration: 40 min Level: Easy Doses: 4 people

Ingredients:

- 2 fennels
- 300 g Catalonia
- 2 anchovy fillets in oil
- 1 orange
- fennel seeds
- extra virgin olive oil
- salt

For the fennel recipe with Catalan sauce, clean the fennel, preserving some of their green, and cut them very finely with the slicer or a mandolin. Then soak them in water and ice for about 10'. Clean the catalogna and cook it in boiling salted water for 2-3', then cool it in water and ice.

Drain the catalogna and blend it in the food processor with the anchovy fillets and 75 g of oil. If you want a very smooth texture, sieve the sauce. Peel the orange alive, collecting the dripping juice in a bowl; cut the slices into small pieces.

Arrange the sauce on the plates, add the fennel and complete with the orange juice and pieces of orange, some of the fennel green and some crushed fennel seeds.

Desserts and Fruit Dishes

Orange braised endive and Grand Marnier

Duration: 30 min Level: Easy Doses: 4 people

Ingredients:

- 2 Belgian endive tufts
- 1 Orange
- Sugar
- Grand Marnier
- Dates
- Grated botargo
- Extra virgin olive oil

Cut the endive heads in half, wash and dry them.

Burn them in a frying pan with a drizzle of oil, placing them on the cut part; cook for 3', turn the salad and sprinkle it just with a little sugar, turn it again and caramelize it for 2-3'; sprinkle it with the Grand Marnier and flame it, then wet with the orange juice and cook it for 5' uncovered and for another 5' with the lid.

Serve half a head of endive each, sprinkling it with grated roe and completing it with small pieces of dates.

Endive with orange juice and black olive powder.

Duration: 1 h 15 min Level: Easy Doses: 4 people

Ingredients:

- 3 tufts of Belgian endive
- 150 g orange juice (2 oranges)
- 60 g pitted black olives
- 50 g butter
- 20 g sugar
- Curcuma and salt

For the endive recipe with orange juice and black olive powder, place the olives on a plate covered with baking paper and bake them in a ventilated oven at 160 °C for 1 hour. Peel the endive, cut each head in half and each half into 3 slices; place them in a saucepan with the orange juice, butter, sugar, a teaspoon of curcuma, a pinch of salt and cook over low heat for 35 minutes.

Take the olives out of the oven and reduce them to powder by chopping them with a knife or blending them. Drain the endive from the cooking sauce and place it on a serving plate. Reduce the cooking sauce over a high flame for about 3'. Pour the sauce over the endive, garnish with olive powder to taste and serve.

Macedonia at the Grand Marnier

Duration: 50 min Level: Easy Doses: 4 people

Ingredients:

- 40 g pistachios peeled
- 2 oranges
- 1 khaki vanilla
- 1 kiwi
- 1 prickly pear
- half-mango
- honey
- orange blossom
- Grand Marnier

For the Grand Marnier fruit salad recipe, peel the slices of an orange, peel the prickly pear and cut the seedless pulp into thin fillets, peel the mango and dice it, peel the kiwi and slice it into slices, then cut the persimmon into slices.

Collect all the fruit in a bowl. Squeeze the other orange and collect about 50 g of juice in a small saucepan with a spoonful of honey. When it boils, remove from the heat and add 2-3 tablespoons of Grand Marnier.

Let the juice cool down, then pour it over the cut fruit, stir gently and leave to marinate for 30 minutes. Spread the fruit in 4 bowls and complete with the roughly chopped pistachios.

Oranges and cream au gratin

Duration: 35 min Level: Medium Doses: 4 people

Ingredients:

- 100 g brown sugar
- 4 eggs
- 2 oranges
- Grand Marnier
- ginger powder
- cinnamon powder
- nutmeg
- vanilla
- icing sugar
- salt

For the recipe of oranges and cream au gratin, peel the oranges and peel the slices. Whip the egg whites until stiff, with a pinch of salt. Heat 2 tablespoons of Grand Marnier and melt the sugar, then let it cool.

Add it to the yolks and whip them until frothy and clear, adding the seeds of half a vanilla pod, a pinch of cinnamon powder, one of ginger and one of nutmeg.

Incorporate the egg whites into the yolks, gently, obtaining a froth. Pour it into 4 ramequins (ø 10 cm). Place the orange slices on top of the cream and bake the ramekins in the oven at 220 °C for 4-5 minutes. Sprinkle them with icing sugar and serve immediately.

Orange frost, green apple and dates

Duration: 3 h 15 min Level: Easy Doses: 4 people

Ingredients:

- 300 g blood orange juice
- 50 g sugar
- 10 g gelatine in sheets
- 16 stoned dates
- 2 green apples
- orange peel

For the orange, green apple and date frost recipe, boil 50 g of water with sugar; turn off, add the soaked and squeezed jelly and let it melt. Pour it into the orange juice and put the mixture to cool in the fridge for at least 3 hours.

Break the jelly with a spoon and put it in the glasses, alternating it with chopped apples and dates. Complete with filleted orange peel.

Almond, orange and carrot milkshakes

Duration: 45 min Level: Easy Doses: 4 people

Ingredients:

- 300 g oranges
- 200 g cereal bread
- 120 g soy milk
- 150 g almonds without peel
- 60 g peeled carrot
- 10 g peanut paste
- Sugar
- extra virgin olive oil
- salt

Cut the carrot into thin strips, then dip them in water and ice for 30' so that they become crispy and curl slightly. Finally, season them with oil, salt and sugar. Blend the soy milk with the almonds, peanut paste and 50 g of water.

To obtain a milkshake with a very smooth consistency, you can pass it through a sieve. Peel the oranges and cut the segments. Keep the juice obtained during this operation.

Slice the cereal bread, toast the slices in a non-stick fat-free pan and dice them. Spread 2 tablespoons of almond milkshake on each plate, a few drops of orange juice, then sit on the orange slices, the seasoned carrots, a diced bread and a drizzle of oil.

Tart with ganache, oranges and cream flowers

Duration: 2 h 10 min Level: For experts Doses: 12 people

Ingredients:

- 480 g sugar
- 200 g flour
- 150 g dark chocolate
- 150 g fresh cream
- 120 g butter6 oranges
- 2 yolks
- creamy ice cream
- vanilla
- peanut oil
- salt and pepper

PREPARATION

Slice an orange very thinly. Prepare a syrup: boil 200 g of sugar and 200 g of water for 5', then remove from the heat. Let it cool, dip the orange slices, drain them and put them on a baking sheet lined with baking paper lightly greased with peanut oil and bake them at 80 °C for about 2 hours.

Cut 4 oranges into slices and then peel them.

Blanch the orange peels in boiling water for 1-2 minutes three times, changing the water each time.

Collect the blanched orange peel and the flesh kept aside (about 400 g in total) in a saucepan with 200 g of sugar. Bring to the fire and cook for about 50 minutes. Keep 2 peels aside, they will serve to complete. Blend the jam.

Mix 120 g of butter with 80 g of sugar, the seeds scraped from half a vanilla pod, a little grated orange peel and a pinch of salt; then add 2 egg yolks and finally 200 g of flour.

Ginger cake with mango

Duration: 1 h 30 min Level: Medium Doses: 4 people

Ingredients:

- 110 g sugar
- 110 g flour
- 100 g butter
- 50 g mango pulp
- 50 g white chocolate
- a chunk of ginger
- 8 g baking powder
- 2 eggs
- a teaspoon of honey

For the ginger mini-cake recipe with a soft mango heart, blend the mango pulp and cook it in a saucepan with honey for 5'. Chop the white chocolate and mix it with the hot mango pulp, obtaining a ganache: let it cool in the freezer for 1 hour or in the fridge until it is firm (about 3 hours).

Melt the butter in a saucepan or microwave. Peel the ginger and grate it. Work the eggs with the sugar with a spoon, then sift the flour and baking powder, then add the butter and grated ginger and put the mixture in the fridge for 30 minutes. Cover with baking paper 4 stencils (ø 6 cm, h 6 cm) and distribute the mixture.

Form 4 balls with the mango ganache, the size of a small walnut, place them in the centre of the mixture and push them gently to make them sink only slightly. Bake the mini-cakes at 180 °C for 12-14', then take them out of the oven and delicately remove them.

CONCLUSION

Thank you for reading this far; I hope it was educational and provided you with all of the skills you need to reach your objectives, whatever they may be.

This book has attempted to bring all of the crucial aspects to the forefront so that you can reap the full benefits of natural products while avoiding the negative consequences.

To produce and use natural antibiotics and antivirals as prevention and treatment of specific diseases, simply follow the information and techniques provided in the book.

In the event that a sickness persists, it is advisable to seek medical advice.

I hope you find this book useful in accomplishing your objectives.

Warning

We urge that you visit your doctor or therapist before beginning any treatment.

www.ingramcontent.com/pod-product-compliance
Lightning Source LLC
Chambersburg PA
CBHW070908080526
44589CB00013B/1229